Wrong Medicine

Wrong Medicine

Doctors, Patients, and Futile Treatment

SECOND EDITION

Lawrence J. Schneiderman, M.D.
Professor Emeritus, Departments of Family and
    Preventive Medicine and of Medicine
School of Medicine
University of California, San Diego
La Jolla, California

and

Nancy S. Jecker, Ph.D.
Professor, Department of Bioethics and Humanities
School of Medicine
University of Washington
Seattle, Washington

The Johns Hopkins University Press
Baltimore

o 643443322

The Johns Hopkins University Press
2715 North Charles Street
Baltimore, Maryland 21218-4363
www.press.jhu.edu

Library of Congress Cataloging-in-Publication Data

Schneiderman, L. J.
    Wrong medicine : doctors, patients, and futile treatment /
Lawrence J. Schneiderman and Nancy S. Jecker. — 2nd ed.
        p. ; cm.
    Includes bibliographical references and index.
    ISBN-13: 978-0-8018-9850-1 (hardcover : alk. paper)
    ISBN-10: 0-8018-9850-1 (hardcover : alk. paper)
    ISBN-13: 978-0-8018-9851-8 (pbk. : alk. paper)
    ISBN-10: 0-8018-9851-X (pbk. : alk. paper)
    1. Medical ethics.   2. Surgery, Unnecessary.   3. Medicine—
Decision making.   I. Jecker, Nancy Ann Silbergeld.   II. Title.
    [DNLM: 1. Ethics, Medical.   2. Medical Futility.   W 50
S359w 2011]
    R724.S3936 2011
    610.69'6—dc22   2010025984

A catalog record for this book is available from the British
Library.

*Special discounts are available for bulk purchases of this book. For
more information, please contact Special Sales at 410-516-6936 or
specialsales@press.jhu.edu.*

The Johns Hopkins University Press uses environmentally
friendly book materials, including recycled text paper that is
composed of at least 30 percent post-consumer waste, whenever
possible. All of our book papers are acid-free, and our jackets
and covers are printed on paper with recycled content.

Do not try to live forever. You will not succeed.

— GEORGE BERNARD SHAW, *The Doctor's Dilemma*

Contents

Preface to the Second Edition ix

Acknowledgments xiii

1 Are Doctors Supposed to Be Doing This? 1

2 Why It Is Hard to Say No 23

3 Why We Must Say No 37

4 Families Who Say, "Do Everything!" 57

5 Futility and Rationing 74

6 Medical Futility in a Litigious Society 89

7 Ethical Implications of Medical Futility 104

8 The Way It Is Now / The Way It Ought to Be:
For Patients 131

9 The Way It Is Now / The Way It Ought to Be:
For Health Professionals 144

10 The High Points: Medical Futility 167

11 Medical Futility: Where Do We Stand Now? 183

Notes 195

Index 221

Preface to the Second Edition

When Johns Hopkins University Press editor Wendy Harris, who skillfully shepherded the first edition of *Wrong Medicine: Doctors, Patients, and Futile Treatment,* invited us to prepare a second edition, we were happy to accept. Since the original publication of our book in 1995, we have witnessed new conceptual, legislative, judicial, and clinical developments that support and extend our original proposals. What we didn't anticipate was the remarkable coincidence of events that occurred as we were writing both editions. Back in 1995, President Bill Clinton was attempting to patch together private health care insurance plans that were excluding millions of Americans and create a new and improved universal health care system. The insurers wanted no part of it, and as a result of powerful lobbying and scary "Harry and Louise" television ads, those efforts disappeared without a trace in a kind of Washington version of the Bermuda Triangle. As we prepare this new edition, another president, Barack Obama, is attempting to overhaul what is, after 15 years of neglect, an even more deranged and neglectful American health care system. His efforts are coming up against, not the stifling stasis of a Bermuda Triangle, but a perfect storm of clamorous Republicans attacking with the lockstep discipline of Roman legionaries, a crashing economy, and a public rendered confused and frightened by a round-the-clock, high-decibel, polarized media.

Back in Clinton's time, we had high hopes that the government would fix the patchwork, irrational, and, worst of all, unjust way Americans were forced to deal with illness. Our hopes were dashed. But as we work on this second edition, they have risen again. Whether or not universal health care coverage will be achieved remains to be seen. Medicine, of course, will move inexorably on, bringing with it many new discoveries and ever more invasive and costly interventions, forcing us to face a host of ethical conundrums—including issues surrounding medical futility. Since publication of the first edition, changes have occurred in four main areas.

Conceptual. We and other bioethicists have published papers addressing the major objections raised by critics. We have emphasized the difference between treatment and care, pointing out that, although a treatment may be futile, care is never futile—a distinction now incorporated in many hospital policies. Also, we have moved our boundary definition of qualitative futility from survival in the intensive care unit to discharge from the acute care hospital, consistent with almost all other published measures of success and failure of life-sustaining treatments. In addition, we have drawn attention to the phenomenon of an aging society, which raises the prospect of abuse of the futility concept. Some might think (wrongly) that a patient's age is relevant to a futility judgment, even when age alone has no bearing on the likelihood or quality of medical benefit. We argue that the concept of medical futility is independent of the patient's age and that physicians should not offer futile interventions to patients, regardless of their ages.

Legislative. Actions taken at the state and federal levels now endorse the right of health care providers and institutions to forgo nonbeneficial treatment. The most prominent example at the state level is the Texas Advance Directive Act, which provides a step-by-step procedure to deal with conflicts, ending in legal immunity for hospitals that choose to withdraw futile life-sustaining treatment. At the federal level, the Uniform Healthcare Decisions Act supports institutions that decline to continue treatment that does not benefit the patient. Many states have signed on to this act.

Judicial. The notorious Terri Schiavo case—involving a vitriolic conflict over whether to maintain or remove the feeding tube of a permanently unconscious woman—seized the attention of the country, and even much of the rest of the world. This case, the longest-lasting litigation in the history of American medicine, presented an anguishing counterexample caused by the failure to apply the concept of medical futility. In another case, the California Supreme Court applied an unrealistic "clear and convincing" standard to overrule a wife's effort to follow the wishes of her severely brain-injured husband to discontinue tube feeding. In their unanimous ruling, the judges commented that if the patient, Robert Wendland, were completely unconscious (which he had been for more than a year), they would not have objected to her decision. Thus, although the man had to suffer for many years in a completely helpless, minimally conscious state before he died, he gave the rest of California a gift of judicial endorsement for the concept of qualitative futility in a permanently unconscious patient.

Clinical. There have been several developments in establishing a standard of practice for medical futility. The American Medical Association has called on all hospitals to record a futility policy and has provided a guideline of step-by-step procedures that lead to permission to withdraw futile treatment. Many hospitals around the country, including the University of California San Diego Medical Center, have documented futility policies consistent with the principles expressed in our book. In San Diego, community consensus has led to a standard of practice. In an important endorsement of quantitative futility, Kellermann and colleagues tested a clinical prediction model against outcomes of out-of-hospital cardiopulmonary resuscitation and concluded that the results were acceptable in accordance with the quantitative proposals put forth in the original paper we published with our colleague Albert Jonsen. One of us (LJS) invited Alexander Capron, a professor of law, who opposed the concept of medical futility, to join in presiding over a conference made up of representatives of more than 20 California hospitals, along with laypersons, lawyers, and judges, to see whether we could define a uniform standard of practice. What came out was even better: the notion of a majority (benefit-based) standard and a "respectable minority" standard that departs from the majority standard. This provides a practical solution to the problem raised by some critics that there is "no universal agreement" about medical futility. For just as we allow some hospitals to refuse to perform abortions, we can accept that a minority of hospitals will disagree that sustaining the life of a permanently unconscious patient is futile. The challenge to the latter "respectable minority" hospitals is that their moral stance imposes an obligation to accept surrogate-requested transfer of such permanently unconscious patients from the majority standard hospitals.

These are only a few of the highlights we describe in these pages. We hope this edition will offer updated insights to colleagues in health care, including medical students, residents, fellows, faculty, and practicing physicians, along with colleagues in nursing, social services, hospice, and health policy. We also hope that our words will reach and prove helpful to a concerned lay public who face choices about health care for themselves and their loved ones.

Acknowledgments

In the first edition of *Wrong Medicine* we devoted a full page to thanking the many colleagues who provided us with opportunities to present and discuss the ideas contained in the book. In the 15 years that have since passed, we have had many more opportunities for discussion and feedback, so many we could not possibly list the names of all those who hosted our presentations for this second edition. You know who you are, and we sincerely thank you. Also, we thank Holly Teetzel, who provided devoted attention to the preparation of the manuscript; London Carrasca, who unearthed hidden references and provided stimulating discussions; and David Strom, who propitiated the computer gods during mysterious digital storms and blackouts. We also thank Nancy Jecker's children, Rachel and Diana, for their patience while she was working on *Wrong Medicine*, first and second editions.

Wrong Medicine

CHAPTER ONE

Are Doctors Supposed to Be Doing This?

More than 20 years before the permanently unconscious Terri Schiavo unwittingly starred in a nonstop cable television circus, the travails of another permanently unconscious young woman made headlines in the daily newspapers and prompted a landmark "right to die" decision by the U.S. Supreme Court.[1] Her name was Nancy Cruzan. While driving home from her job in a cheese-processing factory early one January morning in 1983, the 25-year-old Missouri woman ran her car off a country road and landed face down in a ditch. First to arrive on the scene was a state trooper. He examined the young woman and concluded she was dead. Paramedics arrived an estimated 15 minutes after the accident and immediately set about trying to restore her breathing and heartbeat, which they did after about 10 minutes. But the woman never regained consciousness. By then, her cerebral cortex, the part of the brain that controls the qualities that made the woman Nancy Cruzan—her thoughts, emotions, behavior, memory, capacity to experience and communicate; in other words, all the activities that made her a unique living person—had been irreversibly destroyed. Only the more primitive part known as the brain stem—which controls heartbeat, respiration, swallowing, and peristalsis—

survived, being more impervious to the oxygen deprivation she sustained before cardiopulmonary resuscitation (CPR). Thereafter, Nancy Cruzan remained unconscious for more than seven years, a condition now called permanent vegetative state.[2]

At first, Nancy Cruzan's family, whose members had become active in a head-injury support group, urged physicians to do everything they could to keep her alive—including surgically implanting a feeding tube into her stomach. But three years later, having witnessed the grotesque physical changes such patients undergo, including bloating of the face and stiffening contractures of the arms and legs, they asked the doctors to remove the feeding tube so that she could die in peace. Joe Cruzan, a sheet-metal worker, remembered his daughter as a vibrant, independent, cheerful, active woman who loved animals, children, holidays, and the outdoors. "Nancy would not want to live like this," he pleaded, adding that she would be "horrified at her existence now."

But the doctors and the hospital refused to withdraw the feeding tube without a court order, forcing what was from then on the case of *Cruzan v. Director, Missouri Department of Health* to begin its laborious way to the U.S. Supreme Court. The major obstacle to carrying out the wishes of the Cruzan family was the Missouri Supreme Court, which declared: "The State's interest is in life; that interest is unqualified."[3] It ordered medical treatment to be continued as long as Nancy Cruzan's body held breath and heartbeat. The court acknowledged that it would have allowed her tube to be removed if only she had given "clear and convincing" evidence that she would not have wanted to be kept alive in a permanent vegetative state—a contingency beyond the imagination of most people, not to mention a young, vibrant woman in her twenties.

In a highly publicized decision, the U.S. Supreme Court upheld Missouri's right to apply a "clear and convincing" standard for evidence of Nancy Cruzan's wishes. At the time, this standard was not defined in any legal textbook or statute; rather, it was "left to the sound discretion of the trial court."[4] Yet even though the trial court had been persuaded by the parents' testimony that their daughter would have wanted treatment withdrawn, the trial court's decision was overruled by the state supreme court.[5]

As for Nancy Cruzan, after the U.S. Supreme Court decision, a remarkable change occurred in Missouri's view of the matter. Her friends, whose testimony had never made it to any of the earlier court hearings, reported statements she had made that she would never want to live "like a vegetable" on medical machines. These additional statements were submitted by the family on remand. Ironically, her friends' testimony appeared to impress the state attorney general more than the statements made by her own parents. But by then, many believe, the state of Missouri, embarrassed by the national outrage at the heartbreaking tragedy, was looking for an excuse to withdraw from the case, which it did in the end, concurring with the trial court that "clear and convincing" evidence had finally been produced and allowing the family's petition to be upheld.

It was not exactly the end, though, for even after Nancy Cruzan's feeding tube was removed, carloads of religious zealots descended on the hospital, camped in the parking lots, held prayer vigils, and even tried to force their way in to reattach the tube. But as the Cruzan family said many times, for them Nancy had died back in 1983. "The last thing that we could do for her is to set her free."[6] They finally accomplished that seven years later.

Professor of law George Annas expressed the concerns of many bioethicists at the time: "The case of Nancy Cruzan provides us with a public warning as to how much control we have already ceded the state over our lives, and how far the state has already gone in redefining the 'life' it seeks to 'normalize' and control."[7]

How did medical treatment become such a travesty, such that for the Cruzan family it was not a beneficent healing process but, rather, an unrelenting scourge? Indeed, Nancy Cruzan's condition, persistent vegetative state (which had not even achieved recognition as a diagnostic entity until 1972), could be regarded as having been caused by medicine itself. Her vegetative state was the consequence of brain injury, of course, but her *persistent* vegetative state would not have been possible without sustained medical treatment. Exact data are lacking, but estimates are that between 9,000 and 35,000 permanently unconscious patients are being maintained in hospitals and nursing homes around the country.[8] Until the 1970s and '80s, these patients rarely were kept alive for long periods of time. What accounts for the difference? It is not that medicine lacked the capabilities—for ironically, as in the case of Nancy Cruzan, whose heart, lungs, digestion, and kidneys functioned normally, all it takes is a feeding tube and good old-fashioned nursing care to prevent bedsores and infections.[9] Did financial incentives or fear of litigation suddenly change in the '70s and '80s? Perhaps these are factors, and we will explore them in later chapters. But the principal reason is that maintaining permanently unconscious patients was not considered by society and by physicians to be an appropriate goal of medicine. *Physicians were not supposed to be doing that.*[10]

Why Are Doctors Doing Such Things?

Hospitals no longer consist of silent wards where patients passively wait to recover from whatever ails them under the watchful eyes of doctors and nurses. Rather, they are bustling, high-technology warrens of specialists. Patients are almost always in motion, aggressively propelled in search of a cure, shunted into and out of elaborately equipped suites providing ultrasound, angiography, fiberoptics, radioactive scanning, computerized axial tomography (CAT) and magnetic resonance imaging (MRI), organ transplants, extracorporeal membrane oxygenation (ECMO), laminar air flow, and the by now old-fashioned intensive care units (ICUs), where patients are connected to ventilators, cardiac pacemakers, and a variety of electronic monitors. The impact of all this technology extends well beyond the innovations themselves; indeed, their most important impact may be on the way doctors think. *Technological imperative* is the term used most often to describe this new way of thinking—if "thinking" is the right word: if a means or instrument or medication exists that can produce an effect on a patient's body, then medicine must use it. In short, the instruments of technology rather than patients become the focus of medical attention.

Technological advances, which have brought about incontestable benefits, coincide with the ascending influence of the basic sciences and subspecialties in medical education and practice. Unfortunately, they have caused physicians to fragment their perception of the goals of medicine, leading to an emphasis on the outcomes of discrete parts rather than on the success of the whole.

By contrast, the focus of medical attention throughout the past was always on the patient. Medical treatments, albeit relatively clumsy, either restored health, or yielded to invalid care, or lost the patient entirely. But the goal of the physician was *at the very least* to restore the patient to some level of conscious awareness and participation in the human community—working, living with loved ones, meeting with friends, sharing meals, watching children and grandchildren play, gossiping, arguing, joking, making love. Today, however, there are so many more intermediary stages between health and death, so many more ways to bring patients from the brink of death back to life, sometimes with only partial recovery of body organs—particularly that most sensitive organ, the brain—that we now face ethical problems about the goals of medicine that were unimaginable 40 to 50 years ago. Today patients are being kept alive who cannot experience, much less participate in, the most minimal human activities.

Another new reality about medicine is that it is no longer a private matter involving only the small circle of patient, family, and physician. Today the circle is more like an arena, and there are many witnesses, participants, even intruders. The Cruzan family, after agonizing discussions in the intimacy of their home, came to the conclusion that medical treatment had failed to bring back their daughter. The goal that they and the doctors were striving for had not been achieved. They decided therefore to stop medical treatment. But, as it turned out, the decision was not theirs alone to make. Doctors, nurses, hospital administrators, ethicists, lawyers, judges, third-party payers—all demanded a say. The national media picked up the story, and persons whom ethicist Nancy Dubler dubbed "roving strangers,"[11] activists who seek out such cases for the purpose of dramatizing moral or political agendas, turned the Cruzans' private agonies into a public spectacle.

So, when we question Nancy Cruzan's treatment—Are doctors supposed to be doing these things?—we are actually asking anew the age-old question, What *are* the goals of medicine? Inescapably joined to this question are other questions: Can we as a society agree when treatment fails to achieve the goals of medicine? What are physicians supposed to do and *not* do when treatment fails to achieve the goals we set for medicine? These are the fundamental questions of medical futility. In answering them we will be examining the doctor-patient relationship in the modern era.

Every day, in our view, the traditions and standards of medicine are violated by physicians, nurses, and other participants in medical decisions who fail to reflect about medical goals, or consider that the goal of medicine is not and never has been to offer futile treatment. We emphasize that our use of "goals of medicine" is normative: often a gap exists between the ends that physicians seek and the ends they *ought* to seek. (Here we invoke the multi-layered meaning of the word *ends*, which designates not only goals and purposes but also limits and terminations.)

In short, a desire to restore a vision of medicine's proper ends and reform medical practice is the impetus for this book. Although our central emphasis is to reassert ethical standards for physicians, our arguments carry important implications for other health care professionals and many health care fields. And because medicine as a profession is answerable to society, we contend that restoring this vision will require the active involvement of an educated society. Thus, our book is aimed not only at the medical profession and a specialty audience but at all health professionals as well as the lay public.

Medical Futility from a Historical Perspective

The view of the goals of medicine and medical futility we present here derives from the long tradition of the medical profession. Physicians in classical Greece and Rome saw their efforts as assisting nature (*physis*) to restore health. In the treatise titled "The Art," from the Hippocratic corpus, three roles were prescribed for the physician: alleviating suffering in the sick, reducing the violence of their diseases, and refusing to treat those who were "overmastered by their diseases, realizing that in such cases medicine is powerless."[12] Note that the prolongation of life was not considered a goal of medicine.[13]

Long before discoveries in the fields of cellular pathology or molecular biology, these scientists of earlier days made careful and remarkably accurate observations of signs and symptoms in their patients to determine the natural course of illness. By empirical experimentation with diet and exercise, herbs and extracts, instruments and splints, they saw themselves as allied with the forces of nature, not with supernatural forces. Indeed, to protect themselves from accusations of mercenary greed and charlatanism, they forthrightly acknowledged the limits of their skills and duties. In "The Art" the Hippocratic physician warned, "Whenever the illness is too strong for the available remedies, the physician surely must not even expect that it could be overcome by medicine." The Hippocratic writer further cautioned that a physician should not demand "from an art power over what does not belong to the art, or from nature a power over what does not belong to nature," adding that such ignorance was "allied to madness." Knowing the *limits* of medicine was regarded as an important measure of a physician's skill in integrating the art of medicine and the power of nature. Thus, these early physicians shunned treatments that experience told them were futile and regarded as harmful strenuous efforts to keep an unhealthy, suffering patient alive.

Not until many centuries later, during the late Middle Ages and the associated rise of Christianity in medieval Europe, did medical practice begin to be dominated largely by religion. During this period, medicine took up "prayer, laying on of hands, exorcisings, use of amulets with sacred engravings, holy oil, relics of the saints and other elements of supernaturalism and superstition."[14] At the same time, the Catholic church, which considered abortion, suicide, and euthanasia sins, introduced a new goal for medicine: the prolongation of life.

This new, more expansive view of medicine was reinforced during the scientific revolution of the seventeenth century, when Francis Bacon, for example, defined the goal of science as not merely to "exert a gentle guidance over nature's course" but to "have the power to conquer and subdue her."[15] In other words, scientists began to view science as a power to be exerted *against* nature. We must keep in mind, however, that neither theologians nor scientists, nor for that matter anyone else before the modern era, could ever have imagined life in the many forms in which it comes today, the many states between health and death that are the outcomes of modern medical treatments—for example, Nancy Cruzan's (and Terri Schiavo's) condition, permanent vegetative state.

The classics scholar Darrel Amundsen summarized this evolution and made the following incisive commentary:

> It is well before the advent of modern medicine that physicians were saddled with the expectation that they must do all that they could to cure a patient and they must not desert the patient *in extremis*. Hence, beginning with the late Middle Ages, they were depicted lingering in the background in the death chamber, not able to do anything, but still obligated to be there. The major change since then has been in the increasing capacity of the medical profession to cure disease and prolong life, and the often unrealistic expectations of society that physicians should be able to perform miracles. This has in part resulted from a changed view of nature. Granted, ever since the time of Hippocrates and Plato dispute has intermittently arisen over the question whether the physician works with or against nature in the treatment of illness. Francis Bacon's plea that physicians should seek to prolong life through finding cures for supposedly incurable conditions has blossomed into an attitude that in such a quest it is "man against nature"—the "conquest" of disease involving human ingenuity thwarting nature's purposes.[16]

Later, during the nineteenth century, when medical practice began to profit more conspicuously from the successes of scientific discoveries, it not surprisingly began to pursue more aggressive approaches to treatment. Today we see this combination of religious and scientific impulses survive in casually uttered expressions, such as "life is sacred" and "preserve life at all costs"—high-sounding phrases that have come to dominate medical practice, impelling physicians to pursue even the most futile treatments. But what do we mean by *medical futility*?

Defining Medical Futility

We begin our discussion of the ends of medicine by describing, first, what medical futility is not. *Medical futility* does not refer globally to a patient's situation, to medical treatments in a general sense, or to a person who is ill. The term instead refers to a particular treatment applied to a particular patient at a particular time. We also wish to draw attention to the importance of distinguishing among the terms *treatment, therapy,* and *care.* A particular *treatment* (from the root meaning "to deal with," literally "to handle") may be futile because it fails as *therapy* (from the root "to heal"). Acts of *care* (from the root meaning "to feel compassion for") are never futile.

Medicine's goals are clearly to benefit the person—to restore, to heal ("make whole"). Therefore, they do not include offering treatments that fail to achieve those goals, namely, futile medical treatments. We will devote the remainder of this chapter to presenting and defending a definition of medical futility.

It is important to explain at the outset why a definition of medical futility requires an ethical argument. Unlike definitions of scientific terms, such as *energy* and *mass*, which are part of the discourse of scientists who accept certain scientific theories, the definition of medical futility is not contained in a scientific (or other) theory. Instead, it must rest on a societal consensus that incorporates specific ethical choices—values as well as actions. Just as the modern definition of *death* in terms of "total cessation of all functions of the brain including the brainstem" reflects society's sense of the meaning of human life, so too whatever definition of medical futility society chooses will reflect its conception of the ethical ends and purposes of medicine. Critics have sometimes falsely portrayed our position as one that supports "the supremacy of one group's rights over the rights of another group."[17] On the contrary, we do not support the authority of one group (physicians) over that of another (patients and families). Instead, we support a definition of futility that reflects a consensus process, a process that includes not only physicians, but all health professionals and the broader society. The action of any individual physician must be based on professional standards of care and must be consistent with societal values.

Some have argued that the whole notion of medical futility is too elusive to define.[18] Others have even urged that the term be abolished from the medical lexicon.[19] But as Edmund Pellegrino, former chair of the President's Bioethics Council, pointed out: "Those who call for the abandonment of the concept have no substitute to offer. They persist in making decisions with, more or less, covert definitions. The common sense notion that a time does come for all of us when death or disability exceeds our medical powers cannot be denied. This means that some operative way of making a decision when 'enough is enough' is necessary. It is a mark of our mortality that we shall die. For each of us some determination of futility by any other name will become a reality."[20]

To return to the example of Nancy Cruzan, according to the state of Missouri her feeding tube was not futile because it kept her body alive. So we must start out by asking: Is that the goal of medicine—to keep the body, in whatever condition, alive? Is that what we summon up in our minds when we use the word *life*—the irreversibly unconscious body? Don't we, rather, picture, not a body, but a *person*, someone who is aware of the world around, in touch with it not as a conglomeration of cells and body fluids but as only a specific human being can be—with sensations, thoughts, and emotions? There is no question that the *body* of Nancy Cruzan was alive. It breathed, pumped blood, digested food, excreted. But was that body the *person*, Nancy Cruzan? Was she in possession of the human capacity to experience her own unique life? In short, did she as a person benefit from the intervention she received, namely, tubes delivering artificial nutrition and hydration to her body?

Remarkably, some have tried to reduce the notion of futility to an even more mechanistic and biologically fragmented level. As long as medicine can achieve a physiological effect on any *part* of the body, such as lungs or heart or kidneys, they argue, then treatments such as attempted CPR are not futile.[21] Is this, then, the goal of medicine—to keep an organ system going? Would this satisfy us as a last resort in medical treatment, merely to maintain the flow of air or blood or urine? Most surveys show overwhelmingly that people have other ideas—that past some point in a deteriorating quality of life, well short of merely maintaining organ vitality, they would rather be allowed to die.

Others view futility from the perspective of patient autonomy, arguing that as long as medical treatment can achieve what the patient wants, it is not futile.[22] At first view this would seem a laudable definition of futility. But what if the patient demands surgical removal of unwanted ears, or fingers, or breasts? Or demands that a normal appendix be removed so that he would no longer have to worry that occasional cramps are due to appendicitis? Or demands that doctors carry out cryogenic preservation of her cadaver on the utterly fantastic hope of restoring dead flesh to life? Are there no limits to what medicine owes patients? Clearly there are. Medicine is not a vending machine that dispenses to patients whatever they order regardless of therapeutic benefit. A physician, for example, is not ethically obligated to provide useless treatment on demand, such as antibiotics for a viral infection or laetrile for cancer. And even if the treatment is *not* useless, physicians are still limited in what they may offer. If a patient's goal is to become a world champion bodybuilder with the aid of steroids, the physician is neither ethically obligated nor legally permitted to comply with the bodybuilder's request. A particularly important limitation, in this era of life as a TV movie of the week, is that the physician does not owe the patient a miracle.

Some bioethicists propose that *futility* should refer not just to treatments that cannot benefit patients but also to treatments that provide more harm overall than benefit. The physician-ethicist Howard Brody, for example, argues that anabolic steroids should not be provided to the ambitious bodybuilder because, although they may markedly increase physical prowess for a period of 10 years, they will in the end lead to deterioration followed by death. By calling such a medicine futile, Brody argues, physicians have a way of keeping intact their professional integrity and the ethical standards of avoiding harm to patients. And so, even if prominent athletic associations declared the use of harmful steroids acceptable by their standards, physicians could refuse such requests on grounds of *their* professional standards.[23]

We have a problem with this definition of futility in that its requirements are too weak; it lets too many treatments qualify as futile. We believe that when the ethical decision requires weighing *significant medical benefits* against harms, the responsible adult patient should be allowed to make his or her own decision about treatment. Only when the patient would receive no significant medical benefit from a particular intervention does it become the physician's responsibility not to offer the treatment and, as appropriate, to inform the patient that the treatment will not be offered.

The anabolic steroid is futile not because it harms patients down the road but because it does not provide any medical benefits to patients in the first place. After all, enhancing athletic prowess is not a medical goal; rather, medicine is concerned with restoring health and healing the patient. Giving an athlete large doses of steroids certainly does not make a sick person well, nor does it rehabilitate a disabled person to a level of ordinary functioning. There was a notorious time in recent history when Nazi doctors aspired to make a super race by selectively breeding those they thought possessed superior qualities and exterminating those they thought lacked such qualities. But this goal, which violates the fundamental duty of beneficence to every patient, never has been part of the historical tradition of ethical medicine. Nor does the ethical practice of medicine embrace such a goal today.[24]

It should be clear, then, that the above definitions of the goals of medicine and medical futility are unsatisfactory. The challenge we face is to provide a useful and persuasive alternative definition that not only serves at the patient's bedside but also is acceptable to society at large. For without the informed understanding of an educated and active public, the use of futile medical interventions may continue unabated, with all the irrationalities and painful and costly habits unchanged.

By proposing a definition of medical futility, rather than simply a description or example of futility, we hope to provide the necessary and sufficient conditions for a medical intervention falling under the term. Too often, the everyday understanding of futility in the medical setting is vague, and determining futility is problematic. By saying that the present usage of *futility* is vague, we mean that many people who use this term have not fully thought through its meaning. Yet, a vague term can become more sharply focused when it is more fully specified. For example, *obscenity* is sometimes a vague term. Its meaning becomes clearer, however, when the Supreme Court decides that certain record albums contain obscene lyrics, thus providing substantive information about the meaning of the term. This is analogous to how we intend to proceed with providing a definition of futility. Unlike the legal definition of obscenity, however, the definition of futility we propose must ultimately be consistent with the values of health professionals and the public at large.

We start with a preliminary general definition of medical futility: *Medical futility means any effort to provide a benefit to a patient that is highly likely to fail and whose rare exceptions cannot be systematically produced.* Note first that this definition includes a quantitative component ("highly likely to fail") and a qualitative component ("benefit to the patient"). Note also that the focus of the question when considering medical futility is the patient (derived from the Latin word for "to suffer"), not some organ or physiological function or body substance. Nor is the patient merely any person who has some capricious desire, but a specific kind of person, one who is in particular need of the medical skills and judgment of a physician to alleviate or prevent suffering. Note also that the medical treatment should provide a benefit, not merely an effect. There is an important difference. Medicine is capable of an enormous range of effects that once were unimaginable—adding and subtracting body chemicals, increasing and reducing circulating blood cells, destroying cancer cells, restoring heartbeat, replacing body organs, killing bacteria, subduing viruses and fungi, to name a few. But these effects are of no benefit to the patient unless the patient is capable of appreciating them. The sad fact is that medical treatments could have produced a multitude of effects on the unconscious Nancy Cruzan, but she was incapable of appreciating any of them. Thus, as we will argue, all the treatments aimed at Nancy Cruzan, because they provided no benefit, were futile, and health professionals had no business attempting them.

In reviewing the Cruzan case, it is important that we make clear the reasons underlying our judgment that it is futile to provide life-sustaining treatment to patients like Nancy Cruzan. All patients with complete and permanent loss of consciousness, such as permanent vegetative state, lack a necessary feature of being a person. For, regardless of widely different conceptions of personhood, almost everyone agrees that personhood requires a capacity or potential for conscious awareness. Even some of the most conservative positions about personhood require at least the potential for attributes such as conscious awareness of one's self or one's surroundings, the ability to experience pain and pleasure, or the capacity to interact with others.

Thus, conservatives on the abortion debate argue that at the moment of conception the fertilized egg has the potential to develop these morally important qualities.[25] On the other end of the spectrum are liberal views, such as Singer's utilitarian philosophy, which place emphasis on the individual's capacity to experience pain and pleasure.[26] While most human beings (and many animals) have the capacity for pain and pleasure, those who are permanently unconscious do not experience pain, pleasure, or any other conscious state, nor do they have the potential to do so in the future.

Why is it that even though individuals in a permanent vegetative state would not quality as persons even on the most conservative assessment, we still feel obligated to treat such individuals with dignity and respect? Perhaps this reflects the fact that Nancy Cruzan and others in a permanent vegetative state are past persons. Thus, the emotional attachment that people may have felt toward Ms. Cruzan does not turn off abruptly. Instead, because she is a past person, she has a life story that remains with us even after her loss of personhood and subsequent death. By contrast, debates about personhood that occur in the context of abortion do not raise this issue because the fetus was not a person before conception.[27]

If permanently unconscious patients are not persons, it follows that health professionals have no obligation to attempt treatments to keep them biologically alive, for the subject of ethical obligation is not the biological body but the suffering patient. Although other ethical considerations, such as respect for the patient's dignity and compassion for the family, may lead doctors to provide other forms of treatment, such as anticonvulsants or hygienic care, they are under no duty to offer life-sustaining treatments. Indeed, in subsequent chapters of this book we will make the case that not only are physicians not obligated to offer futile treatments, they *should not* offer futile treatments.

Now it might mistakenly be argued that the mere fact that a permanently unconscious individual is a living member of our species suffices to show that that individual is a "person" and therefore is an appropriate subject of medicine. However, it is important to distinguish carefully between "person," which carries moral connotations, and "human being," which is used in its descriptive biological sense. As philosophers use the term, *person* refers to a being, potentially of any species, who possesses the qualities that are necessary and sufficient for possessing fundamental moral rights, including a right to life. Hence, if permanently unconscious patients are not persons, then by definition they lack a right to life and are not owed the medical means necessary to stay alive. Once again we point out that neither late medieval theologians nor seventeenth-century scientists who advocated life-prolongation were familiar with living human beings who lacked the capacity to ever recover consciousness (even if severely impaired). Nor were they likely to have imagined the notion of "life" that can be preserved in such a discordant state by present-day technology.

It is worth noting that some who agree that human beings in a permanent vegetative state lack the moral qualities necessary to qualify as moral persons, with a right to life, will argue that all forms of human life (both personal and nonpersonal) possess intrinsic value. For them, even nonpersonal forms of human life possess special value (or, in religious terms, "sanctity" or "sacredness"), and therefore there is some merit to preserving them.

We sympathize with the humane impulse behind this argument but respond that even if one thought that human life in any form was intrinsically valuable, it hardly follows that it is *medicine's* job to attempt to preserve all forms of human life. Medicine's focus has never been (and, we maintain, should never become) the biological organism as such, but is the suffering *person* (i.e., patient). Thus, even though physicians may have a responsibility to treat human life—from the earliest stages of conception to brain death—with dignity and respect, only persons are proper subjects of life-sustaining medical interventions.

To draw an analogy, nearly everyone agrees that a "brain-dead" individual (i.e., dead by whole brain criteria) is a past person, and as such the physical remains should be treated with respect; however, a "brain-dead" individual is no longer seen as a *patient* or an appropriate subject of life-sustaining *medical* treatment. In other words, even though a "brain-dead" individual may continue to have living human cells, it is not a living person. This marks a crucial turning point in how practitioners of medicine view it. Once a patient meets the criteria for death by whole brain criteria, medical apparatus, such as respirators and artificial fluid and hydration, are withdrawn. Likewise, we are arguing that an individual in a permanent vegetative state is a past person, whose biological remains should be treated with dignity and respect. However, it should not be medicine's task to use the means at its disposal to keep the physiological processes of such an insensate individual running indefinitely on demand.

Further Defining Medical Futility: Its Quantitative Aspect

One thing every medical student learns is "never say never." This is the problem of uncertainty in medicine. Quantitative probabilities can never be precisely determined. Clinical circumstances are so complex that one can never be absolutely certain of the outcome. Indeed, philosophers since David Hume have pointed out that the very notion of causality is suspect. As Hume noted, we never directly observe the "causal glue" that connects two events. Instead, "the mind goes beyond what is immediately present to the senses" to infer a causal relationship.[28] The philosopher Karl Popper emphasizes that science can never produce knowledge that is certain. Even after we fail a million times to resuscitate a cadaver—drawing the not unreasonable conclusion that the dead cannot be revived—how do we know the next effort will not result in success? It would take only one success to falsify the conclusion drawn from all the previous experiences.[29] In medicine, for example, we have no way of knowing with certainty that a treatment causes an effect to occur in the body. We observe only that on numerous occasions the application of this kind of treatment precedes bodily changes. We *infer,* on the basis of probability, that the treatment is the responsible (causal) agent. It is important to make this point clear: Medical practice almost never achieves certainty; rather, it depends on empirical clinical experience. Physicians prescribe specific drugs and dosages because such treatments are observed to achieve beneficial effects (or more beneficial effects than harmful effects) often enough that they feel confident these practices will work in the future. But each individual patient represents a new challenge: will the particular drug and dosage work on this particular patient in this particular circumstance? Uncertainty lurks ineluctably in the shadow of every medical decision.

Today, as more and more therapeutic options are available, this struggle with uncertainty leads to a kind of paralysis of action. If the physician can never be absolutely certain, then isn't the physician obligated to do anything and everything that *conceivably might* work? This paralysis of action expresses itself in a relentless momentum. Once high-technology machines are started—which *conceivably might* work—they are almost impossible to stop. But the world is full of tales of miraculous events, up to and including the raising of the dead. Physicians have never been obligated—or even expected—to reproduce all the miracles of mythology. That is what we mean by "rare exceptions [that] cannot be systematically produced." At most, physicians can do their best to "assist nature" in the real world. To overcome this paralysis of action in the face of uncertainty, we pose the following commonsense question: *Because we can never say never, can we agree that if a treatment has not worked in the last 100 cases, it would be "reasonable" to conclude that it is futile?* We propose this then as our specific and practical definition of the quantitative aspect of medical futility.

Although we present a specific proposal, we recognize that people may disagree about exactly where the threshold for futility should be. For example, some may think that waiting for 100 failures before acknowledging a treatment's futility sets the threshold too low, while others may contend that the threshold is set too high. All would probably agree with the more fundamental idea that *at some point* the likelihood of medical success is so poor that attempting to achieve it is futile. (A well-known definition of insanity attributed to many savants, including Einstein, is "doing the same thing over and over again and expecting a different result.")

But what about those who do not agree, who refuse to accept *any* notion of futility? For example, what about the person who argues: If I'm willing to pay for it, why can't I have life support for my loved one's permanent vegetative state as long as I want? Or what if a religious group expresses the belief, based on a biblical precedent, that resurrection is possible and demands that the dead bodies of its adherents be preserved with mechanical ventilation, cardiac stimulation, and intravenous fluids?

In response, we first point out that physicians' professional responsibilities prohibit them from providing a treatment solely because someone is willing to pay for it. As we will emphasize often in this book, the goals and limits of medicine are not determined merely by money. Medicine, as a profession, is distinguished by the goal of healing patients. If it were to be practiced solely to satisfy the whims of those who would pay, the ethics of medicine would become indistinguishable from those of the "oldest profession." Therefore, any proposal to permit medical consumers to obtain different levels of treatment above a "decent minimum" depending on their willingness to pay still must remain within the limits of the appropriate goals of the health care profession: medically beneficial care. And just as no health care plan allows physicians to provide steroids to athletes willing to pay for the drugs, no plan should authorize physicians to provide futile treatments to those patients willing to pay higher premiums.

As for the second objection to futility based on religious or cultural beliefs, we will address this subject at greater length in Chapter 7. Here we will briefly note that in our pluralistic society, religions and cultures with specific beliefs that impinge on medical practice are not free to impose those beliefs on others, although they are free to form their own medical provider systems that provide and pay for such practices. In practical terms we suggest that the solution to this conflict for medical providers and the public may lie in recognizing not only a majority standard of care but also a standard of care embraced by a "respectable minority" of hospitals.[30]

Interestingly, a consensus already seems to be forming in the medical community about the application of our quantitative notion of futility. At the same time we were developing our original quantitative proposal, studies appeared evaluating CPR in a variety of patients, ranging from very-low-birthweight babies to elderly patients to patients with metastatic cancer to patients rushed to the emergency department after experiencing irreversible cardiac arrest outside the hospital. Independently, the research physicians at different medical centers came to the same conclusion: Even though attempted CPR occasionally produced a few hours or even a few days more of life in the hospital, the procedure was futile, because it failed to result in hospital discharge in more than about 1 in 100 of these patients.[31] Thus, neither the probability nor the quality of the outcome was regarded as fulfilling the goals of medicine.

Recently, Sasson and colleagues applied our quantitative guideline as the standard to evaluate a formula called the Basic Life Support Rule (BLS) for predicting outcomes in cases of refractory out-of-hospital cardiac arrest. After analyzing the results of a large empirical study, these researchers concluded that "the BLS rule had a positive predictive value for predicting lack of survival, which is within the acceptable range used by medical ethicists for defining futility."[32]

Further Defining Medical Futility: Its Qualitative Aspect

In *The Republic,* Plato wrote: "For those whose lives were always in a state of inner sickness Asclepius [a mythical demigod-physician] did not attempt to prescribe a regimen . . . to make their life a prolonged misery." And "a life of preoccupation with illness and neglect of work isn't worth living."[33]

Unfortunately, as our technological skills have become more powerful and the technological imperative has become more compelling, "prolonged misery" has afflicted many who fall by the wayside while hoped-for miracles are pursued. The misery, however, and the costs and suffering involve not only the treatment failures. What about those for whom treatment is considered a success? In the past, a successful treatment was not so dubious or problematic. Inevitably, the patient appreciated it as a benefit. Can we say that of Nancy Cruzan, as she lay in her unconscious state, with her cerebral cortical tissue atrophied and replaced by fluid? She experienced nothing—certainly no benefit from her survival. Nor would she ever. Thus, we must consider a qualitative aspect to medical treatment. In other words, we must distinguish between an *effect* and a *benefit.*

As we have already said, treatment of a patient such as Nancy Cruzan in permanent vegetative state is by definition futile because she is incapable of experiencing, much less appreciating, anything that is being done to her. We would argue also that the goal of medicine is not to keep people alive in the

ICU, where they are *preoccupied* (to use Plato's word) with treatment and can do nothing else with their life. Such patients are there because they require constant and close attention as well as immediate access to physicians, nurses, and technicians who can diagnose and treat medical crises. They cling to life by machines designed to blow oxygen into their lungs, machines designed to monitor body fluid balance and blood chemicals, and still other machines designed to sound shrill warnings while initiating and controlling heartbeat by repeated electric shocks. When they were developed in the 1960s, ICUs were intended to be only temporary havens for desperately ill patients who were expected either to die or to recover. But today, ICUs represent a kind of purgatory for many patients, who remain for months and months on the brink of death before succumbing to their illnesses. Such patients are totally dependent on intensive medical care for survival—in the ICU. Is this a goal of medicine, to sustain life in the ICU? We believe not.

Furthermore, we ask, is it a goal of medicine to sustain life indefinitely in an acute care hospital? In the modern acute care hospital, as in the ICU, patients are preoccupied with treatment and must devote their energies to sustaining, rather than living, their lives. In light of this, we propose that the definition of futility apply to life-sustaining treatments where the outcome is that patients will never leave the acute care hospital. This proposal expands the boundary of medical futility beyond what we proposed initially in the first edition of *Wrong Medicine* and reflects the general consensus that *hospital discharge* is a measure of successful outcome.

Consider, for example, the futility policy of the University of California San Diego Medical Center, which is the model for many area hospitals. It defines *futile treatment* as "any treatment without a realistic chance of providing an effect that the patient would ever have the capacity to appreciate as a benefit, such as merely preserving the physiologic functions of a permanently unconsciousness patient" or any treatment that "has no realistic chance of achieving the medical goal of returning the patient to a level of health that permits survival outside the acute care setting of UCSD Medical Center." The policy goes on to state that in the event of disagreement among the parties involved in the treatment of a patient, futility will not be invoked before the completion of an appropriate dispute resolution process, which it outlines.

Immediately following the medical futility policy is a statement of the Medical Center's policy on comfort care, which is defined as "care whose intent is to relieve suffering and provide for the patient's comfort and dignity. It may include analgesics, narcotics, tranquilizers, local nursing measures, and other treatments including psychological and spiritual counseling. It should be emphasized that although a particular treatment may be futile, palliative or comfort care is never futile."

Thus, our specific and practical definition of the qualitative aspect of medical futility: *If a patient lacks the capacity to appreciate the benefit of a treatment, or if the treatment fails to release a patient from total dependence on the acute hospital setting for survival, that treatment should be regarded as futile.* We reiterate that care aimed at relieving suffering or maintaining the patient's dignity should be offered to all patients.

Again, not everyone may accept the threshold we have chosen for qualitative futility. Nevertheless, everyone can agree that, as Dr. Pellegrino states, "some operative way of making a decision when 'enough is enough' is necessary. It is a mark of our mortality that we shall die. For each of us some determination of futility by any other name will become a reality." In other words, at some point the quality of medical outcome may become so poor that it is futile.

Physicians are beginning to reevaluate not only their duties and obligations but also their limits. This is an important first step. Ultimately, society at large will have to express agreement clearly: The ends of medicine lie not with mere biological survival nor with the patient imprisoned within machines and tubes. At the very least, the ends of medicine require providing the patient with the capacity to participate in the human community. And although this level of participation can be minimal, common sense would dictate that it does not refer to insensate bodies or patients irrevocably immersed in a hospital's life-support machinery. We strongly advocate patient autonomy and the right to make medical treatment decisions over a wide qualitative range— and there are many noteworthy examples of people who have achieved remarkable satisfaction despite severe physical or mental disabilities—but we draw a line *at some point* between patients' rights to choose their own quality of health and life and the medical profession's obligations to achieve those ends. Limits should be clearly stated: Patients can demand of medicine help in maintaining any quality of life they like so long as that life is not irreversibly unconscious or confined to the ICU or the acute care hospital setting, for these are beyond the goals of medicine. At the very least, the goal of medicine should be to make it possible for patients to survive outside such settings. On the other hand, we wish to emphasize a point we have already made: A particular *treatment* may be futile, but *care* is never futile; nor is a *patient* ever futile. The second, qualitative dimension of futility provides a sufficient condition for a treatment counting as futile. In other words, if an intervention meets this criterion, that is all that is needed to show that it is futile.

Taken together, the quantitative and qualitative standards we propose for medical futility provide the necessary and sufficient condition for medical futility. Each criterion is sufficient by itself to confer medical futility, yet meeting one or the other of these criteria is necessary.

In what follows, we will address all of these points in more detail. In Chapter 4 we emphasize the importance of continuing to offer comfort care to the patient and emotional support to the family after futile interventions are stopped. In Chapter 5 we distinguish between withholding treatments on the basis of futility and withholding treatments on the basis of rationing. The medical profession does not owe every treatment imaginable; but until society establishes a policy of rationing that applies just limits to medical treatments, the medical profession's responsibility is to advocate for any treatment that provides medical benefits to patients.

Ironically, there is an unexpectedly positive consequence to forcing physicians and patients to acknowledge medical futility. Instead of continuing the useless repetition of unsuccessful treatments, physicians will be spurred to search for more beneficial treatments. In fact, this is the goal of evidence-based medicine. An honest acknowledgment of futility, in our opinion, will make medical progress and discovery more likely rather than less likely.

The Mythical Power of Futile Treatment

Until now we have refrained from the obvious, that is, stating the dictionary meaning of *futility*. In the *Oxford English Dictionary* the word is defined as "leaky, vain, failing of the desired end through intrinsic defect." The word derives from the ancient *futtilis,* a pot, wide at the top and narrow at the bottom, that was used in religious ceremonies on behalf of Ceres, the goddess of fertility, and Vesta, the hearth goddess. Because of its narrow base, the futtilis tipped over whenever it was filled. Although the futtilis was useless for everyday tasks, as a religious vessel it played a powerful role in mythic drama. The philosopher Don Postema asks, "Can a medical treatment similarly be useless from one point of view, but have mythic significance from another perspective? What cultural meanings do futile therapies carry?"[34]

Postema goes on to point out that Sisyphus has always been seen as a symbol of futility, being condemned to Hades to eternally roll a rock up a hill, only to see it roll down again. "However," Postema adds, "Albert Camus in the 'Myth of Sisyphus' takes the character and life of Sisyphus as an emblem for the modern age, a hero in an absurd world. Sisyphus is a tragic figure because he is conscious of his task; he knows that what he is doing is futile, yet he persists in its performance."[35]

Postema thus reminds us of the importance of symbols. We must ask, Does the pursuit of futile treatment serve some need of patients for heroic action? Does it satisfy some deeply felt cravings in an antiheroic age? Does it offer a magical alternative to the mundane world of cause and effect? One of the realities of contemporary society is that medicine has for the most part replaced religion as a source of spiritual meaning, consolation, and miraculous expectation. Many treatments, such as attempted CPR, have become rituals in the mind of the public, conveying religious and mythical power. Is it in answer to these deep spiritual needs that patients and families sometimes demand futile treatments? Are these life-saving treatments misguidedly taken as measures of caring and compassion? Images of abandonment are frequently heard and words such as *starvation* and *neglect* used to describe dying patients who are not connected to intravenous lines or gastrostomy tubes or ventilators or assailed with efforts at CPR. Sadly, however, futile interventions are not good ways to promote caring and compassion. Often they are obstructive and harmful. All too often, they make a mockery of caring by substituting invasive procedures for human communication and touch, only adding to patient discomfort in the terminal stages of disease.

In pursuing our concept of futility throughout this book, we hope we have not lost sight of the spiritual needs of a modern society, where many have lost faith in religion. Good physicians often call on priests, ministers, rabbis, and other spiritual leaders for help in caring for their patients. But the reverse also has occurred, particularly in the last few decades: patients and families look to medicine and science for miracles, rather than looking to religious sources. In the past when people sought a miracle, they went to church and prayed to God. Now they go to the hospital and demand it of the doctor. In other words, they expect, or even demand, that doctors perform miracles by saving their loved ones from the brink of death, even though accomplishing this exceeds the physician's powers and is beyond the point of reasonableness.

Medicine has not been an unwilling collaborator in this deception but has taken advantage of the public's infatuation with "miraculous breakthroughs," "miracle drugs," and other hyperbolic claims. Indeed, physicians may at times be flattered by the public's esteem and by its tendency to put the doctor on a pedestal and liken the physician to God. It was inevitable that medicine would be held to account, so now it is not uncommon for members of the clergy and judges and politicians to support highly emotional (and often well-publicized) demands of patients and families for outcomes that are beyond the capacities of medical practice, not to mention science. However, as the medical ethicist Albert R. Jonsen reminds us: "The public and physicians alike are affected by the symbols of life saving and life sustaining technologies. But these symbols can be deceptive when they reach beyond the reality. The reality is that medicine does have real but limited efficacy. Refusal to admit futility into the picture of medicine's efficacy is to honor the symbol rather than the reality. It deceives patients and the public rather than educating them and enhancing their autonomy. Far from depriving patients of autonomy, the appropriate invocation of futility reveals the genuine options that persons have when they seek help from modern medicine."[36] It is this distortion of the goals of medicine that led to the tragedy of Nancy Cruzan.

As David Rothman, a professor of social medicine and history, argues, the most important issues today have "nothing to do with budget or with concern for the common will, but with the recognition of futility, a desire to prevent pain, and an acceptance of the inevitable."[37]

In the next chapter we will explore why it is so hard to accept the inevitable and say no to futile treatment. But first, a word about the approach we will take throughout the book. Although presenting opposing perspectives, we clearly intend to make a case for our own. Like law professor Ronald Dworkin, whose superb work, *Life's Dominion,* addresses abortion and euthanasia, we make no apology for pursuing an extended argument rather than depositing in your hands a bland on-the-one-hand-on-the-other-hand tome. Indeed, we hope that the reader will find "an example of a now neglected genre: an argumentative essay that engages theoretical issues but begins with, and remains disciplined by, a moral subject of practical political importance."[38]

CHAPTER TWO

Why It Is Hard to Say No

Ethics consultations take many forms. They range from nocturnal phone calls from resident physicians worried about the legal risk of accepting a patient's request for a Do Not Attempt Resuscitation (DNAR) order, to bedside discussions in the intensive care unit (ICU) with distraught or resigned patients, to strained and lengthy conferences involving every combination of patient, families, doctors of varying specialties, nurses, psychologists, social workers, lawyers, and hospital administrators. Inevitably, intense emotions become interwoven with philosophical reflections, activities in the human repertoire that moral philosophers have traditionally tried to keep apart. By the time we are called to assist in a medical decision, there is rarely an obvious "right" answer. The situation is beyond a simple fix. Instead, the ethics consultant, together with the health care team, face options that are charged with irrational hopes at best, intolerable outcomes at worst. And yet so often, by the time we are called, decisions have already been made to press on with certain treatments, despite a general acknowledgment that the better choice would have been an entirely different approach. Why does this happen? Why is it so hard to say no to treatments that are clearly providing no benefit and are only pro-longing suffering?

Alicia M. was a 14-year-old girl who had leukemia. The disease had relapsed several times over the past few years despite chemotherapy. Even though Alicia was legally a minor, the medical team was impressed that she had a full understanding of her illness and treatments. As her condition took a decisive turn for the worse, she began to express a preference for narcotics and other measures that would maximize comfort as opposed to chemotherapy, antibiotics, and transfusions, treatments aimed at prolonging her life. But her parents, avid bodybuilders and physical fitness buffs, kept urging her not to give up. They persuaded her and the medical team to attempt a bone marrow transplantation despite the low odds of success. This treatment required ablating her immune system first with total-body irradiation and chemotherapy. Her postoperative period was punctuated by several near-fatal episodes of shock and sepsis. Finally, she developed large areas of open, painful, and easily contaminated skin wounds and required a ventilator to assist her breathing.

Prodded by the nurses, the doctors finally agreed among themselves that continuing ventilator treatment in these circumstances was futile and that Alicia had no realistic chance of overcoming her present condition. All they were doing was prolonging her suffering. After consulting with one of us to gain reassurance about ethics and the law, the physician in charge of Alicia's care presented the facts to the family. He strongly urged that Alicia be kept comfortable with sedation and narcotics and be allowed to die without any further efforts at resuscitation or life-prolongation. The parents resisted at first, then agreed. But as they sat by their sleeping daughter's bedside and watched her breathing become weaker and more irregular, they abruptly changed their minds and demanded that vigorous measures be reinstituted to treat her faltering heart and blood pressure and assist her breathing and combat infection. So fiercely did the parents express themselves that the doctors relented and resumed aggressive measures at life-prolongation, placing Alicia back on the ventilator and starting IV medications to stimulate her heart, raise her blood pressure, and combat infection. But these measures served only to keep her alive and miserable three more days. For months afterward, in the dining room, in the nursing stations and corridors, in fact almost everywhere doctors and nurses gathered, the young girl was the subject of anguished discussions. Why had they let that happen? Why had it been so hard to refuse the demands of Alicia's parents for treatments all the health providers had come to agree were futile?

In this chapter we briefly present some of the reasons for the difficulty in saying no that we have encountered in our clinical ethics work. In later chapters we discuss them in more detail. Some of the factors are inextricably linked to the human psyche; some reflect our contemporary medical culture and the training of physicians and nurses; others arise out of "real-world" legal and political considerations.

Human beings resist death. This fact is so self-evident that we consider it unnatural—pathological—when a person seeks to die. A physician who is confronted by a patient expressing suicidal thoughts is most likely to make a diagnosis of severe depression, seek to assess the immediate risk, and either attempt treatment or call on a psychiatrist to manage the patient. Physicians are even granted legal authority in most states to take control of patients who are judged to have a mental illness and likely to harm themselves and can hospitalize them against their will. This is evidence that society assumes that normal, healthy people would resist death and only deranged people would not. Indeed, preferring death over life is seen not only as irrational but also as sinful by many segments of society. Yet a patient might wish to live *but not in an intolerable state.*

Thus, one reason it is so hard to say no to futile treatment is because society's life-protecting propensities are so strong: its first impulse—and the impulse of medical providers—is to keep life going at all costs. In the case of Alicia's parents, this attitude contained an even more powerful component. They took pride in challenging their bodies, and experienced pleasure and enhancement of their self-image when they could triumph over pain and physical limits. For them, life seemed to possess even greater value when it was death-defying. Although this heroic view of life is in many ways admirable, it became a terrible curse when projected onto another human being, their daughter, whose illness and suffering had led her to a different view of life.

Human beings have difficulty accepting their humanity. Philosopher Martha Nussbaum suggests that the difficulty we have in accepting the limits imposed by our mortality is that such acceptance requires a kind of heroism. In her rich and perceptive essay "Transcending Humanity," she draws attention to the moment in the wanderings of the mythological Odysseus when he rejects

Calypso's offer to settle down. She has tempted him with immortality and ageless love. Odysseus acknowledges that his wife, Penelope, is far beneath the beautiful goddess in form and stature: "She is mortal," he admits, "you are immortal and unaging."[1] Yet, even so, the long-suffering sailor opts to continue his voyage, thus choosing "not only risk and difficulty, but the certainty of death; and not only death, but the virtual certainty that he will at some time lose what he most deeply loves, or else will cause, by his own death, great grief to her. . . . He is choosing the whole human package: mortal life, dangerous voyage, imperfect mortal aging woman. He is choosing, quite simply, what is his: his own history."[2]

Referring to the ancient Greek concept of hubris, Nussbaum goes on to say, "There is a kind of striving that is appropriate to a human life; and there is a kind of striving that consists in trying to depart from that life to another life. This is what *hubris* is—the failure to comprehend what sort of life one has actually got, the failure to live within its limits (which are also possibilities), the failure, being mortal, to think mortal thoughts. Correctly understood, the injunction to avoid hubris is not a penance or denial; it is an instruction as to where the valuable things *for us* are to be found."[3]

In medicine, hubris tempts patients and physicians to strive to exceed medicine's limits and ask for everything, even the impossible. Yet when a humanly meaningful life is no longer possible, the better course is to follow Odysseus's model: to choose our own history with humility and dignity.

Physicians have difficulty accepting the limits of their power. Physicians, too, have a corresponding hubris. As the ethicist Daniel Callahan observes, the modern era of medicine has transformed death from a biological or natural evil to a moral evil and medical failure, as though an amendment had been added to the physician's Hippocratic oath: "If we do not use our newly available technologies to save lives, we can be held accountable for the loss of those lives."[4] This transformation in our attitudes toward death occurs from the very beginning by medical education and the socialization of medical students. It is reinforced every day by medical practice, which takes credit for saving life and blame for failing to do so. Rather than regarding death as our common and inevitable fate, or locating our own mortality within nature's cycle of birth and death, medicine has come to view death as its enemy to conquer. Rather than admitting the possibility that certain states of existence are worse than death, medicine tends to imagine that death always represents the worst kind of evil empire.

These assumptions must be examined anew to make room for the idea of medical futility and a more realistic appraisal of medicine's limits. Medicine's basic commitment is not to life in any form, but to the patient, the "suffering person." Therefore, a patient's death, though always a *loss*, is not necessarily a *failure*. Indeed, a "good" death, as viewed by the physician-ethicist Howard Brody, should be "hailed as a medical success story." Brody reminds his colleagues that "all our patients eventually die, and it is wrongheaded to see death itself as a sign of medical failure. Rather, we should acknowledge failure when the ravages of disease or ill-constructed medical interventions produce a 'bad' death."[5] And one of us (LJS) often repeats this idea on ICU rounds after questioning the physicians, "How did the patient die?" by reminding them, "If a patient dies, it is not necessarily a medical failure. If a patient dies badly, it *is* a medical failure."

The physicians treating Alicia's leukemia had at their command a vast array of treatment possibilities, including powerful (and toxic) chemicals that destroyed her leukemia cells (along with many other kinds of cells) and antibiotics to attack viruses, bacteria, and fungi. They even had a capability that several decades ago was no more than a scientific hope based on promising experiments in mice—a technology that made it possible to replace the very marrow in her bones. Because of the seemingly limitless powers at their disposal, Alicia's physicians probably grew accustomed to the idea that they always had something more they *could* offer. Yet the *ethical* question is whether they *should* offer these interventions, whether they are good for the *patient*. Rather than encouraging humility, which the moral philosopher Karen Lebacqz calls "a sense of one's limits . . . one of the goods internal to the practice of health care,"[6] their technological skills and treatments may well have lured the physicians into a technological imperative: if it can be done it should.

Worse, the tools at medicine's disposal may encourage a delusion of omnipotence. This sense of power resembles that of a gang lord accustomed to carrying a concealed gun. The weapon represents for the gang lord not only power, but his very identity. The hardest thing for the gang lord would be to go out in the streets without his weapon. The hardest thing for some physicians is to face the family of a dying patient without some new technological offering, thus undermining a hard-gained sense of self-worth. Yet the kindest approach would be to acknowledge that there is no treatment that can save their loved one's life, and add, "Now we will do everything to help her to live

and get the most out of her last days and die with as much comfort and dignity as possible." Sadly, it is much easier for many physicians simply to attempt a new futile treatment, making a show of intense commitment to the
patient as a way of convincing observers that they are using their powers to
the fullest.

Not surprisingly, it was the nurses, rather than the physicians, who were
the first to show genuine understanding of Alicia's condition. By her bed con-
stantly and perceiving that her drawn-out existence would be wracked with
pain and suffering, the nurses realized that continuing to apply life-saving
interventions would be a cruel and uncaring response. Perhaps they saw that
the ventilator's primary goal had become one of comforting the family and
the physicians, not the patient.

Further, forcing Alicia to be entirely preoccupied with receiving medical
treatment, so that she could not even communicate meaningfully with family and
friends, condemned her to live her last weeks of life banished from the human
circle of family and community. In the past, such a banished existence—
exile—was imposed as punishment for capital crimes and considered worse
than death. Perhaps Alicia's nurses recognized better than her physicians that
a life apart from the web of relationships and projects that fasten a person to
the human social world was in its own way a state worse than death. Such a
state of banishment, whether it consists of unremitting pain and suffering or
perpetual unconsciousness (or even worse, possible minimal awareness as suggested by functional MRI observations in a few patients who nevertheless are
condemned to perpetual, helpless immobility and incapacity to interact with
the environment), cannot be regarded as a beneficent goal of medicine.[7]

Everyone has struggled so hard, we can't give up now. Sarah J. was a seven-
month-old girl who had congenitally abnormal lungs and received a lung
transplant at one of the country's leading medical centers. For months following the surgery, Sarah never left the hospital as the doctors struggled to keep
the child alive, despite increasing evidence that the congenital condition af-
fecting her lungs involved other organ systems as well. Soon it became apparent that the child was doomed to die, but because the physicians had worked
so hard, and the child (and the child's parents) had suffered so much, no one
had the heart to call it quits. Only when a military reassignment forced the
parents to move and transfer the child to a different hospital were they put in
the hands of new physicians who felt no such emotional burden. To these
physicians the futility of continuing with various life-preserving interven-

tions was clearly apparent. A conference was arranged with the family, physicians, nurses, and an ethics consultant. Painful facts were laid out and discussed frankly and sympathetically. Confronted with this fresh approach, the parents reevaluated their feelings and soon agreed to let their daughter die without any further suffering.

Such problems with the intense and sometimes rocky course of organ transplantation are not uncommon. Post-transplant care involves the most sophisticated weapons in the technological arsenal and can be an emotional roller coaster, with miraculous survival waiting at one end and death buried within tubes and machinery in an isolated laminar flow room at the other. Physicians, patients, and their families become locked in a mutual dependency, relentlessly pursuing more and more desperate and futile measures to keep the patient alive—including even repeated efforts at transplantation— because of the momentum that has developed. Yet the facts are harsh. If a first heart or liver or lung transplant fails, a second effort in the wake of the failure has a much poorer chance of success.[8] At this time the approximately 100,000 patients who are waiting desperately for their first chance at such organs and dying at the rate of 9,000 a year would almost certainly have better results. But when asked about the apparent irrationality of performing repeat organ transplant operations despite the sharply reduced odds of success, surgeons will almost always point out how emotionally difficult it is to "abandon" a patient once the process has begun. "Everyone struggled so hard, we just couldn't give up."

Why is everyone miraculously rescued but me? In an eloquent passage from her novel *Death Comes for the Archbishop,* Willa Cather described the "solemn social importance" of death in an earlier era:

> In those days, even in European countries, death had a solemn social importance. It was not regarded as a moment when certain bodily organs ceased to function, but as a dramatic climax, a moment when the soul made its entrance into the next world, passing in full consciousness through a lowly door to an unimaginable scene. Among the watchers there was always the hope that the dying man might reveal something of what he alone could see; that his countenance, if not his lips, would speak, and on his features would fall some light or shadow from beyond. The "Last Words" of great men, Napoleon, Lord Byron, were still printed in gift-books, and the dying murmurs of every common man and woman were listened for and treasured by their neighbours and kinsfolk.

These sayings, no matter how unimportant, were given oracular significance and pondered by those who must one day go the same road.[9]

Today, patients who learn they have an incurable illness are more likely to feel only isolation and betrayal. All around them, it seems, another lucky soul is displayed on the evening news, having been rescued from the brink of death by miraculous drugs, virtuoso operations, and the latest scientific discoveries. Small wonder that many of those who expect no such triumphant outcomes feel ignored and cast aside amid the celebrations of modern medicine. To die is perceived not as an inevitable final chapter, a moment to be treasured and done right, but as an avoidable mishap—if only the person had the strength of character to hang on a little longer until the hoped-for miracle drug came along that allowed one to do away with, or at least put off, death. Death, in this secular age, is rarely promoted as an opportunity to pass "through a lowly door to an unimaginable scene," from this vale of tears to the bosom of God.

Juzo Itami, the Japanese filmmaker, provides a poignant commentary:

> Traditionally, when people were about to pass away they stayed at home surrounded by the people close to them. The dying person was the central actor. People had this idea of a gallant death done with deep bravery. People around them accepted the fact that this person is about to pass away and communicated with them. There was a culture of death. People now use science. Science means the defeat of death. They no longer want to look death in the face. Death is worthless, scary, like something you flush from your house. You take this person to the hospital because you don't want this thing to happen in your house.[10]

Is it any surprise that few people can look with equanimity on their impending death? In fact, the very words "culture of death" are rattled ominously by the same zealots who denounce efforts to support frank and compassionate end-of-life discussions between physician and patient as "death panels." Faced with this kind of environment is it not much easier—for both patient and bystanders, including the physician—to forge ahead with treatment, any treatment, even useless treatments? To do less would be to reject science, to surrender in battle, to prefer a worthless, scary thing to one's own life; and even worse, to suffer the belief that one lacked some essential ingredient of character and was thereby judged by fate as undeserving of one of the many miracles granted to so many others.[11] Anyone who has experienced or sympathized with or imagined the death of a loved one in these terms can understand how saying no to medical treatment—any treatment, anything at all—could become a virtually unthinkable option.

Bystanders feel compassion and guilt. Almost every doctor who cares for seriously ill patients has had the following experiences: After long and agonizing discussions, members of the patient's family finally decide to limit or forgo aggressive, life-prolonging treatments for a loved one and instead emphasize comfort care. Suddenly, an estranged relative flies in from a distant state and expresses outrage that the person she has not seen for years is being so cruelly and callously neglected. Or a child lies permanently unconscious after being discovered face-down in a backyard swimming pool, the cerebral cortex irrevocably destroyed. The air is filled with cries of blame or guilt. Someone neglected to lock the gate or watch the child closely. The only possible expiation is to keep the unconscious child alive, using every imaginable machine or drug; for as long as the child lives, one can cling to the hope that a miraculous recovery will take place and all will be forgiven. Nor is this phenomenon limited to patients' families. Sometimes physicians who have caused a disastrous outcome, either through bad luck or error, insist on keeping the patient alive despite the utter bleakness of the condition and prognosis. For them, to allow death is to admit failure or, even worse, fault.

A compassionate physician will not "do everything" if all that means is attaching the patient to one more piece of invasive technology rather than doing everything possible to alleviate the patient's suffering. Compassion means literally "suffering together with another, participation in suffering" and "when a person is moved by the suffering . . . and by the desire to relieve it."[12] Compassion goes awry when self-deception leads a well-intentioned health professional to think that applying futile treatments will relieve a patient's suffering by achieving a miraculous cure. Alternatively, compassion is ill-informed when a well-meaning doctor or nurse feels that the only way to relieve the patient's suffering, show caring, or keep hope alive is by indiscriminately using all possible means at medicine's disposal.

A compassionate response to a patient's or a family's request for futile interventions is open communication, in which the health professional seeks to understand the reasons and motivations for the request. Only then are doctors and nurses well prepared to align themselves with patients and families, validate the patient's and family's feelings, and explain what medicine can do to help. Unfortunately, the impersonal nature of modern medicine leads many health professionals to turn reflexively to high-technology fixes (meticulously "following the numbers" of laboratory tests), while underestimating or deriding the importance of low-technology care and ongoing communication. In the modern era, open-ended communication about feelings is not something physicians feel they have time for. It makes some physicians uncomfortable because it seems inefficient, rather than being directed toward discrete goals. Whereas technological methods are precise and measurable, conversation in which patients and family members express feelings and fears is open-ended and imprecise; it requires the health professional to relinquish control during the encounter and perhaps to feel personally sad, disturbed, and vulnerable. To "participate in suffering," as compassion requires, demands health professionals to resist the tendency to deploy futile methods and instead feel emotional pain and turmoil in response to the patient's pain and suffering. The compassionate doctor or nurse thereby acknowledges a common humanity with the patient.

The prospect of a child's death is viewed not only with grief but also with a sense of injustice. As described at the beginning of this chapter, many of us who conduct ethics consultations learn that it is especially difficult to let a child die. More than the death of an elderly person, death in a child is seen as premature, cruel, and unjust. The sociologist Frederic Hafferty showed that physicians-in-training have particular difficulty accepting the death of younger patients. "Students were not only more likely to feel that the terminal status of these [younger] patients was unfair, but they were also more likely to assume that the patients must feel the same way."[13] By contrast, the students in Hafferty's study were urged in their training to view death in the elderly patient as "something they needed to learn from" and "move beyond." It should come as no surprise, then, that doctors often feel a greater obligation to continue futile treatments for young patients, as though such persistence compensates for fate's unfairness. The consequence of these attitudes is twofold:

> *Overtreatment:* If we regard the death of a small child as a greater evil, we may go to greater lengths to try to prevent it, using life-saving measures that are futile and not in the patient's best interest.
>
> *Undertreatment:* If we regard the death of an old person as relatively acceptable, we may decline to use treatments that would benefit the patient.

Both of these responses are ethically unsupportable. After all, the fact that death's timing influences our feelings and attitudes does not suffice to show that death is objectively worse, or that our feelings are justified and should be acted on. A better approach is to understand life not as something we are "owed" a fair share of, but as a gift or benefit we are fortunate to have. Then a proper attitude toward the death of a child is not that the child did not get what she deserved, or had a right to, but instead that we are grateful for whatever time the child had.

It is worth noting that the view that death is worse when it befalls a young person does not seem obvious or true to people living in other cultures, nor has it seemed so to people living in other times. As the philosopher John Kilner observes, the Akamba people of Kenya regard death in old age as worse than death early in life, believing that "the older a person becomes, the more intricately interwoven that person becomes in the lives of others, and the greater the damage done if that person is removed. At the same time, the older person has wisdom—a perspective on life that comes only with age—which is considered to be a particularly important social resource."[14]

Similarly, the great playwrights of ancient Greece and Rome regarded death in old age as tragic, while treating the death of a younger person as beneath tragic dimensions. Only adult men—indeed, according to Aristotle, only persons renowned and of superior attainments, such as rulers and heroes—were considered to have sufficiently deep feelings, a great enough capacity for suffering, to be worthy subjects of tragedy. Their misfortunes, therefore, were of great consequence. Children, by contrast, were generally regarded as too innocent and unformed to be capable of great suffering themselves. Their impending deaths evoked profound compassion principally for the adults whose suffering such deaths caused. In Euripedes' play *Medea,* for example, Medea murders her children (offstage); nevertheless, the playwright directs the audience's sympathy toward the pain and suffering felt, not by these children, but by Medea herself, who acted out of revenge, and by Jason, their father. Imagine a made-for-TV movie today treating children so offhandedly!

The philosophical literature from this time offers a somewhat different twist. According to the philosopher Epicurus, "Death . . . , the most awful of evils, is nothing to us, seeing that, when we are, death is not come, and, when death is come, we are not."[15] In other words, death should not be considered an evil for anyone, because it leaves us immune from future harm. Epicurus argues:

1. What makes the loss of something bad is that someone suffers.
2. Once we die, whatever happens no longer causes us to suffer.

3. Then death leaves us immune to future harm.
4. It follows that neither the mature man nor the young child is harmed by death once it has occurred.

Yet regardless of how much our attitudes have changed since ancient times, no matter how much we treasure or even favor children over adults or elderly people, there is still no reason to pursue futile treatments in persons of any age. The reason is that futile treatments, by definition, do not benefit the patient. Using a ventilator in a patient who is in a permanent vegetative state is futile and should not be done regardless of whether the patient is 8 years old or 80. Judgments about the benefit or futility of treatments require honest assessments of outcomes in particular patients, not sentimental or stereotypic group comparisons.[16]

Caregivers may fear lawsuits if they fail to offer treatment. In addition to all the factors noted above, there are practical "real-world" legal and political reasons that it is difficult to say no to futile treatment. Ninety percent of physicians acknowledge that they fear the legal consequences of forgoing treatment and will even admit their well-known tendency to practice "defensive medicine."[17] As we will discuss in Chapter 6, many physicians hold distorted and exaggerated beliefs about their legal obligation to continue or offer futile treatments. In our ethics consultations we attempt to deal with legal risks in a measured and realistic way. One potent statement we repeat as often as necessary: only one physician has ever had a criminal conviction for deliberately (as opposed to negligently) allowing—or even causing—a patient to die. He was Dr. Kevorkian, the notorious "Dr. Death," who was exonerated numerous times by juries for acts of assisted suicide he openly admitted he had performed and was successfully put in prison only after the television show *60 Minutes* aired a videotape he had provided that showed him defiantly performing voluntary euthanasia. Despite the rarity of legal prosecution and conviction, the fear of facing trial is nevertheless pervasive, and however ill-founded that fear is, physicians often would rather plow ahead with futile treatments than risk being sued.

Physicians fear adverse media attention. Physicians confronted by angry family members over controversial treatment decisions may consult the hospital attorney. Some hospital attorneys, of course, will properly advise the physician to provide whatever beneficial treatments the patient wants or whatever treatments are in the patient's best interest. But, as these disputes unfold, it

often becomes painfully clear that the attorney's client is neither the physician nor the patient but the hospital. Pressured by the attorney and "risk managers," the hospital in turn might pressure the physician to continue inappropriate treatments as a way of avoiding adverse publicity. And sadly, it is true:
in today's world, public relations are best maintained by pursuing, rather than
forgoing, treatment, even if treatment is clearly ineffective and futile, and
even if it prolongs the patient's suffering. Public relations receive priority over
ethical deliberation and a genuine and serious application of the law. Families
or other parties demanding futile treatments may even increase pressure on
the hospital and medical team by threatening not only to call their lawyer but
also to contact newspapers and television stations.[18]

Insurance influences treatment. Families find it easier to demand, and hospitals find it easier to accede to requests for, treatments that are financially painless. An insurance policy that covers continuing treatment on the ventilator
for a patient who will never leave the ICU makes continuing such futile treatment much easier for all to justify. Hospitals feel no disinclination to accept
reimbursement; and patients and families tend to feel ethically entitled to the
futile treatment because it is covered under their insurance plan. Yet this approach, which cedes authority and responsibility to insurance companies, is
wholly untenable. Physicians and others cannot ethically absolve themselves
of the duty to help the patient and do no harm.

Desperate people deserve anything they want. One of the forces at work when
physicians continue to attempt futile treatment is that patients or families
make desperate pleas for help. The easiest way to deal with desperate persons
is to give them what they want. This force has reached even the highest level
of government and become health policy. Activists for diseases such as AIDS
and Alzheimer's persuaded the Food and Drug Administration to change its
approval policy and expedite the provision of drugs on a treatment basis before they were proved to be beneficial. Even now, advocates for the expedited
provision of drugs argue that certain conditions are so serious or lethal that
patients who have these conditions are entitled to any treatments they want—
even possibly useless and harmful drugs.

Although we sympathize with the desperation motivating these patients
and their advocates, we feel a sense of despair as well. Sanctioning dubious
drugs before their therapeutic efficacy is established by careful clinical trials
only *delays* the discovery of useful drugs. Because only a rare few drugs that
initially look promising ultimately turn out to be beneficial, most patients

with these conditions will almost certainly experience *more* suffering with their disease as well as with deleterious drug side-effects. Many patients will be deceived into thinking that the drugs provided under medical auspices might be more beneficial than they really are. As the ethics and legal scholar George Annas cautioned: "The excuse that patients who are dying with treatment and 'have nothing to lose' will not do. Terminally ill patients can be harmed, misused and exploited."[19] Moreover, while demanding treatments that may well be futile for themselves, such patients are also depriving future patients of the possibility of swift progress in discovering new treatments.

All of the above factors—psychological, cultural, legal, economic, and political—influence medical practice today and must be clearly recognized. Whether or not readers agree with our specific descriptions, they will surely understand the larger implications. If we as a society can find so many reasons *not* to accept "a kind of striving that is appropriate to a human life,"[20] *not* to admit to the possibility of futile medical treatment, then physicians will have little incentive to ever shift away from aggressive life-saving procedures toward beneficial and caring alternatives.

CHAPTER THREE

Why We Must Say No

Rarely had one of us seen the medical team look so beleaguered. Hunched around the conference room table, the nurses, interns, residents, social worker, and attending physician—a bright, well-read, and compassionate woman new to the faculty—all conveyed the same message: We're trapped. The medical record they handed over, only the latest of a number of volumes, was several inches thick. Mrs. Boxley (not her real name) was a 92-year-old woman transferred to the hospital from a nursing home because of high fever and suspected pneumonia.

It was already her fourth hospitalization this year, which was still some months from being over. Mrs. Boxley had an affliction not uncommon to elderly people, angiodysplasia, a recurrently bleeding malformation of the blood vessels lining her large bowel. Two of the hospital admissions had been for surgical procedures to save her from dying of massive hemorrhage. The other two hospitalizations—like the current one—had been to treat her for episodes of pneumonia resulting from aspiration of food and secretions.

The medical team's gloom was precipitated by circumstances that seemed to be beyond their control, decisions made by the previous team caring for the woman. Those past decisions were forcing them to do things now that made no sense. For example, it was becoming evident that Mrs. Boxley had severe dementia, not only when she was sick with pneumonia or recovering from surgery but even when she was as healthy as she could be. Descriptions by her nursing home attendants indicated that, though not unconscious, she seemed to derive no satisfaction or pleasure from her existence. The only sounds she made were grunts and cries of discomfort and pain. Over the last year it had become almost impossible to feed her without causing her to gag and cough and of course to aspirate food into her lungs. Yet whenever a nasogastric feeding tube was laboriously inserted through her nose, she cried out even more and pulled it out. This time, the nursing home director made clear, she would not take the woman back unless the doctors secured a gastrostomy tube through her abdominal wall directly into her stomach. Because Mrs. Boxley had left no advance directive regarding the treatments she would want under these circumstances and had no relative or friend who could speak on her behalf, the previous medical team had concluded that they had no choice but to comply.

By the time we arrived at the bedside, the feeding gastrostomy tube was in place, the pneumonia was resolving, and the woman was moaning and crying with all her restored strength. Clearly Mrs. Boxley was not deriving any benefit from her treatment. "But what can we do?" the doctors protested. "The decisions already have been made. We're trapped."

As is often the case, the hospital nurses caring for the woman were the first to demand the ethics consultation. What they were being ordered to do simply made no sense. They were having to pump into her body liquefied nourishment she could not even taste, suction her trachea, clean up her incontinent wastes, and monitor her vital signs in readiness to leap in with everything from drugs to support her intermittently falling blood pressure to rib-cracking attempted CPR in the event her heart stopped. These acts violated their most fundamental impulses of compassion, not to mention their professional obligation, to alleviate suffering and provide comfort. At first, they aimed their comments angrily at the physicians who had ordered them to carry out the daily tasks. But the physicians threw up their hands. They *agreed* with the nurses. If it had been up to them, they would write a Do Not Attempt Resuscitation order and emphasize comfort care. But what could they do?

As we went around the conference room table, we confirmed to everyone's satisfaction that each person there—physician, nurse, social worker—was of the same mind, that because of the patient's condition she was incapable of experiencing any benefit from the treatments aimed at keeping her alive, particularly the gastrostomy tube. In other words, all the health providers caring for Mrs. Boxley considered these treatments futile. All sensed they were participating in something terribly wrong—yet they kept doing it.

What was wrong, we suggested, was that the health providers were failing to recognize that they were not obligated to provide futile treatments. And it was up to them to say no.

How common is this scenario of doctors pursuing treatments they don't believe in? All too common, it seems. Mildred Solomon and colleagues surveyed 687 physicians and 759 nurses in five different hospitals. Almost half of the providers and almost three-quarters of the doctors admitted that they had acted "against their conscience" in pursuing aggressive treatments on terminally ill patients.[1] How many Mrs. Boxleys were among them?

As we emphasized earlier, the goal of medical practice is not to provide any treatment imaginable but to serve the best interests of the patient by providing *beneficial* treatment. Holding physicians responsible for drawing the line at nonbeneficial, that is, futile, treatment has the effect of demarcating patient rights, but it protects them from abuses as well.

Up to now we have taken the position that treatment decisions offering a benefit should respect patients' wishes: patients are entitled to choose or refuse any such treatments. But in this chapter we will qualify that argument by pointing out that patients' wishes must be situated in the broader context of family and community needs and interests, not limited to but certainly including practical economic considerations. In other words, sometimes health providers (ethically) must say no.

The Border between Patient Autonomy and Physician Authority

Ethicists and a consensus of court decisions, including the previously cited U.S. Supreme Court *Cruzan* decision, have made it clear: Tube and intravenous feeding and hydration are to be regarded as medical treatments which, like any other medical treatments, can be stopped under appropriate circumstances. As the ethics consultants in Mrs. Boxley's case, we recommended that, of course, if she had any relatives or friends involved in her care, the doctors should try their best to get them to understand that the tube feeding was providing no therapeutic benefit. For their own peace of mind, it would be preferable for them to accept and be part of the decision to withdraw it. But ultimately it was up to the doctors to say no.

The doctors listened and agreed, but it soon became apparent they still were not happy. The tube was already in place. We might have been able to say no *before* it was inserted, but we can't just pull it out *now* . . . can we?

The answer, we said, is yes—once again, if the treatment is not significantly benefiting the patient. In both law and ethics, withholding and withdrawing treatments are regarded as equivalent acts. If the treatment is not indicated, that is all that matters: stopping is the same as not starting. Granted, doctors and nurses may feel that, psychologically, it feels different to remove an intervention that is already in place than it does to withhold from intervening in the first place. Yet, in the United States, from both moral and legal standpoints discontinuing tube feeding, or "pulling the plug" on a mechanical ventilator, for example, is regarded as no different from discontinuing any inappropriate medical treatment. Nor does it matter whether the treatment is hand-delivered out of a bottle of pills, squirted through a syringe, or propelled by electrical power. As expressed in the influential California Appellate Court decision, *Barber v. Los Angeles County Superior Court,* "Each pulsation of the respirator or each drop of fluid introduced into the patient's body by intravenous feeding devices is comparable to a manually administered injection or item of medication. Hence, 'disconnecting' the mechanical devices is comparable to withholding the manually administered injection or medication."[2]

The *Barber* decision had been announced in 1983, almost 10 years before Mrs. Boxley's medical team brought their plight to the ethics consultant. Since then, the decision has been cited innumerable times in high courts around the country as one of many precedents for withdrawing unwanted and futile treatments. During the decades of the 1980s and 1990s, medical and nursing associations, along with bioethics groups, began formally taking positions and recommending that futile treatments be withheld, or be withdrawn if they were already under way. Thus, the President's Commission for the Study of Ethical Problems in Medicine and Biomedical and Behavioral Research (1983), the Hastings Center (1987), the American Nurses' Association (1988), the American Academy of Neurology (1989), the Society of Critical Care Medicine (1990), the American Medical Association (1991, 2009), the American Thoracic Society (1991), and the American Heart Association (1992) came out in favor of limiting medical care that is no longer beneficial to patients. Perhaps the earliest statement came from the President's Commission. In its 1983 report, *Deciding to Forego Life-Sustaining Treatment*, the commission cautions that "the care available from health care professionals is generally limited to what is consistent with role-related professional standards and conscientiously held personal beliefs. A health care professional has an obligation to allow a patient to choose from among medically acceptable treatment options . . . or to reject all options. No one, however, has an obligation to provide interventions that would, in his or her judgment, be counterthera-peutic."[3] Subsequent statements explicitly recognize the term *futility* and caution physicians against applying futile interventions.

Yet even for sophisticated physicians in an academic medical center, it was as though these events had never happened. As we have already seen and will see again in this book, medical treatments continue to be imposed and demanded in ways that lack any ethical support and defy common sense.

As Solomon and colleagues observed to their chagrin, most of the 687 physicians they interviewed "were uncertain about what the law, ethics, and their respective professional standards say on this matter [withdrawing treatment]. In addition to this uncertainty, the interviewed respondents reported being less likely to withdraw treatments than to withhold them for a variety of other reasons, including psychological discomfort with actively stopping a life-sustaining intervention; discomfort with the public nature of the act, which might occasion a lawsuit from disapproving witnesses even if the decision were legally correct; and fear of sanction by peer review boards."[4]

We have already seen how health care providers, courts, and politicians, lacking a true understanding of the obligations of the medical profession and its limits as well as its powers, ran roughshod over the reasonable demands of the Cruzan parents to free their daughter from being maintained through medical means in a state of perpetual unconsciousness. In Chapter 6 we will see that in some court cases, the pressure for futile treatment came from the other side, the family. In one situation, the husband of Helga Wanglie persuaded the court to compel doctors against their judgment to continue life support on his wife, who had been in a permanent vegetative state for more than a year. In another case, the mother of Baby K demanded that repeated emergency life-saving treatment be carried out on her daughter, who was born without most of her brain, a condition known as anencephaly. And, of course, there was the notorious case of the permanently unconscious Terri Schiavo, whose parents launched a prolonged battle over the status of a feeding tube that involved the courts, the state legislature, Congress, even the president of the United States.

In all such instances, medicine was viewed as a force to be exercised on demand, rather than judiciously and selectively directed at illness. Unfortunately, we are beginning to see the consequences of this view. For although the powers of modern medicine can inspire awe, it is increasingly apparent they also can arouse in the public a contrary view: an inordinate fear of being trapped by a dehumanizing technology with no hope of escape.

One startling bit of evidence for the pervasiveness of this latter view was the popularity of a do-it-yourself suicide book published by the Hemlock Society, an advocacy group supporting voluntary euthanasia.[5] Astonishingly, when the book came out it was an immediate bestseller and grist for widespread pontification. What could possibly be so appealing about an instruction manual for taking one's life? The answer to this question seems to be a deep distrust felt by many individuals toward physicians. Patients worry, Will my doctors make humane and compassionate end-of-life decisions? Or will they ignore suffering and force on me unwanted technological indignities? These people—and they seem to number in the many thousands—are apparently drawn to the idea of taking their lives (and their deaths) into their own hands. In other words, as a result of Nancy Cruzan and other highly visible cases, medical treatment has come to be viewed by many as an unleashed menace rather than as a beneficent healing process.

Blame for this state of affairs is passed out freely. Some point to physicians and the entire "medical-industrial complex" which, for venal or misguided moral reasons, insist on perpetuating life-preserving treatments to absurd extremes. Others find fault with patients and families, who, while striving for miracles or heroic actions, demand unrelentingly that "everything be done." The fact is, our pluralistic society—through courts and legislatures—has not yet agreed on a coherent set of values to effectively counter extremes from either side.

But this may be changing. Since the publication of the first edition of *Wrong Medicine*, a great deal of activity has taken place in medical organizations, the courts, and the legislatures with respect to medical futility. We describe below a few of the legal events, summarized in an excellent review by law professor Thaddeus Mason Pope.[6]

Pope notes that a majority of states have now passed statutes directed at allowing physicians to refuse to provide futile treatments. He cautions, however, that the terminology employed (e.g., "significant benefit," "medically inappropriate") may be too vague to reassure physicians. "Because providers are unsure how to satisfy the standards for legal immunity, they remain reluctant to unilaterally refuse requested treatment."[7] Texas is an exception, although its precision rests in procedures rather than definition. The Texas Advance Directives Act (TADA), provides a series of explicit, legally prescribed sequential actions to resolve intractable disputes. If the health care providers, after following all the prescribed procedures, still cannot gain agreement from the surrogate for withdrawing what the physicians deem to be inappropriate life-sustaining treatment, the physicians may withdraw the treatment with immunity from disciplinary action and from civil and criminal liability.[8] According to Pope, "TADA is widely perceived to be a successful model to follow. Consequently, it is no surprise that other states have been looking to copy it." Noteworthy also is that the statute has resisted many efforts by ideological opponents to overturn it.

We have one concern with TADA, however. We believe that an institution not only must define a set of procedures, but also must put forth clear definitions and ethical justifications for pursuing those procedures. This concern is shared by Dr. Edward Pellegrino, former chair of the President's Bioethics Council, who argues: "To establish a procedure for a decision, after all, is to recognize implicitly that something must be decided in an orderly way. The procedure itself is only a means. Unavoidably, it must turn on some set of criteria for action."[9]

Pope reminds us that there are two contrasting approaches to the courts: *ex ante*, which seeks judicial action to permit or prevent a medical decision *before* it is carried out, and *ex post*, which seeks the court's judgment *after* the medical decision has been carried out. Application to the courts can be initiated *ex ante* by either the provider (seeking declaratory relief or permission to stop treatment) or the surrogate (seeking an injunction ordering the provider to continue the treatment). An *ex ante* application is usually a misguided tactic for the health care providers. Why? "Judges have never relished deciding life-and-death medical treatment cases"; hence, they typically grant temporary restraining orders and preliminary injunctions to maintain the status quo. A lengthy lawsuit inevitably follows, during which time, Pope observes, the patient usually dies. As a result, "few courts ever ultimately addressed the underlying core merits of futility disputes."[10]

Contrary to what happens when physicians seek *ex ante* permission from the courts before making a medical decision, in *ex post* cases physicians with only rare exception prevail after the withdrawal of treatment they deem inappropriate—in other words, if they act and then defend their action. Other than the blatant Kevorkian exception, the rare exceptions are those in which "the provider's non-consensual refusal was so secretive, so insensitive, or so disrespectful as to constitute the intentional infliction of emotional distress."[11] Such behavior should be condemned, of course, whether or not the treatment is futile. As Pope says, "Providers are rarely sanctioned for careful, considered refusals of life-sustaining medical treatment. In contrast, they are regularly sanctioned for negligently or recklessly refusing it."[12]

What of the future? Is it possible that the medical profession and the public will continue on the path to recognizing the necessity to forgo futile treatments? Not surprisingly, we are optimistic. As we have discussed above and discuss further in Chapters 8 and 9, much of what we describe here has already ignited a debate among physicians about medical futility. It is our hope that the second edition of this book will bring even greater attention to the subject and foster critical discussion not only among members of the health care and legal professions, but also in society at large.

Money

One obvious reason society must begin to resist inappropriate and nonbeneficial medical treatment is that it can no longer afford to waste valuable resources. As George Lundberg, former editor of the *Journal of the American Medical Association,* stated more than a decade ago: "We Americans value health, and we don't mind spending a lot of money for it. But we want value for our money, and we are currently convinced that, as a nation, we are not getting our money's worth. This must change."[13]

Dire warnings of spiraling health care costs are reported almost daily in the media. Already our country spends more than 17 percent of its gross domestic product on health care, almost double the percentage spent in Great Britain and well above that of every other civilized country in Europe as well as Canada. Furthermore, those countries provide insurance coverage for everyone, whereas in the United States over 40 million people lack health insurance. Not only are health care expenditures already high, they are increasing at a rate of 12–15 percent a year, about four to five times the rate of economic growth. The cost of the current U.S. health care system is $2.5 trillion a year, amounting to more than $6,000 per person.[14]

Many factors contribute to the rising cost of health care. They include the proliferation of expensive, high-technology medical equipment; the aging of the population; the focus on "rescue medicine" rather than public health and other preventive measures; and the increasing use of costly treatments for illnesses such as cancer, AIDS, and heart disease.

Given the above, it is ironic and insupportable to apply costly, nonbeneficial medical treatments to insured Americans, while at the same time denying even the most basic medical services, including preventive screening or prenatal care or management of chronic diseases such as diabetes, to the uninsured. Many Americans support a right to basic medical care; no one has seriously argued that insured Americans have a right to futile interventions. This irony is not lost on the physician-ethicist Paul Farmer and colleague Nicole Gastineau Campos, who note that in affluent areas where bioethics has blossomed, bioethicists are asked to address the quandary ethics of individual patients, such as "elderly patients for whom further care may be deemed futile, even though the machine of 'care' grinds on, leaving family and providers feeling a bit ground up themselves; other 'high tech' tertiary care-driven issues abound." By contrast, in poor regions futile interventions are not foisted on insured populations. "These are not, to say the least, the urgent medical ethics questions in resource-poor settings."[15] Not only can futile interventions, which benefit no one, be invasive and harmful to patients; they can also be wasteful and detrimental to society: fewer resources are left to provide beneficial services to poor and uninsured patients, who go without. This approach to medical care is detrimental to the health of populations while offering no counterbalancing benefits to individual patients. The continued insistence on futile interventions for *insured* individuals is even more irrational in the light of our country's failure to guarantee the most basic care to *uninsured* Americans.

For a while there was hope that the environment would substantially improve under the Obama administration as physicians and health care researchers made an effort to educate the public about "comparative effectiveness research" as part of health care reform.[16] This concept was described in a report to the president and the Congress by the Council of the American Recovery and Reinvestment Act (ARRA):

> Patient-centered comparative effectiveness research focuses on filling gaps in evidence needed by clinicians and patients to make informed decisions.
> Physicians and other clinicians see patients every day with common ailments,

and they sometimes are unsure of the best treatment because limited or no evidence comparing treatment options for the condition exists. As a result, patients seen by different clinicians may get different treatments and unknowingly be receiving less effective care. Patients and their caregivers search in vain on the internet or elsewhere for evidence to help guide their decisions. They often fail to find this information either because it does not exist or because it has never been collected and synthesized to inform patients and/or their caregivers in patient-friendly language. When they do find information it may be informed by marketing objectives, not the best evidence. . . . This research is critical to transforming our health care system to deliver higher quality and more value to all Americans. . . . One private citizen unaffiliated with any health care group summarized, "It is more important than ever to engage in robust research on what treatments work and what do not."[17]

As Alvin Mushlin and Hasan Ghomrawi state, "In this era of high-tech care, there is little likelihood that less-complex and cheaper therapies will emerge as preferred approaches, unless CER [Comparative Effectiveness Research] is allowed to lead to the identification and validation of such treatments."[18] The authors then go on to point out that such research shows that old, familiar, inexpensive diuretic medications to treat hypertension prevent heart attacks more effectively than expensive, heavily promoted, and more commonly prescribed drugs.

Sadly, special interest groups have already persuaded Congress to exclude any examination of costs and banned using such research to "mandate" changes in Medicare, as well as to allow industry representatives (who promote and profit from the more expensive drugs) to distort the strict conflict-of-interest rules to ensure that science is free of inappropriate commercial influence.[19]

However that issue is resolved, there is still a further step we as a society will have to address. While making first-order choices, namely, how much to spend on health care overall, we will also have to make some second-order decisions, namely, choosing areas within health care to reduce expenditures, thereby saving resources for other areas of health care. As we indicated in the previous chapter and will discuss in Chapter 5, it is not enough to view the problem merely as cost containment and rationing. Making choices on these grounds will be time-consuming and difficult for society. But as we wait for the process to go forth, are we really willing to forsake other vital needs in order to pursue futile treatments? As we have pointed out, if certain treatments offer no reasonable chance of providing a benefit, they simply should not be attempted. Even if in the future every American had insurance coverage and access to health care, it would not be morally supportable to offer patients futile treatments. Even if insurance would pay for these treatments, they fail, by definition, to meet the test of helping the patient.

To take but one example, in 1994, the Multi-Society Task Force estimated that the number of adult and pediatric patients being kept alive in permanent vegetative state at 14,000 to 35,000 at a cost of between $1 billion and $7 billion per year.[20] (Extrapolating from European studies, Bernat accepts a still very large but lower prevalence estimate for the United States of about 9,000 patients.)[21] A 1988 survey by the Hastings Center estimated that keeping a patient in a persistent vegetative state alive consumes $126,000 to $180,000 per year. Although these costs and burdens on families and the medical care system are striking, it is important to note that what we are dealing with is not a rationing or cost-containment issue, but rather a *misuse* of medicine itself. The reason to forgo life-sustaining interventions in patients in persistent vegetative state is not that such interventions are expensive (which they are), but rather that they do not benefit the patient.

By contrast, if we assume 3,000 to 4,000 patients with failing hearts (about a third of whom would be expected to die while waiting) and only about 1,500 potential donor hearts available each year in a region served by heart transplant centers, this is not a question of futile medical treatment but rather a difficult problem in making choices. The choice may be one of cost containment—perhaps on the whole we would rather reduce the number of heart transplant procedures and use the money saved for other worthy treatments. Or it could be a rationing problem in that we decide to make use of all the available donor hearts, allocating them according to some criteria that may combine medical as well as social characteristics. In both cases it is important that we not complicate the issue unnecessarily by spending money and resources uselessly on futile treatments. These should be eliminated from the ledger of obligations to maximize the availability of treatments that do work.

How does all this apply to Mrs. Boxley? It is perhaps fruitful to contrast our view with that of the ethicist Daniel Callahan. In his book *Setting Limits,* Callahan proposes that "after a person has lived out a natural life span"—which would "normally be expected by the late 70s or early 80s"—"medical care should no longer be oriented to resisting death."[22] Thus, by his criterion, the

92-year-old Mrs. Boxley would no longer be eligible for life-saving medical technologies. But what would Callahan do about her feeding tube? Apparently he would continue to use it to keep her alive because he is opposed to withdrawing artificial nutrition and hydration. Following Callahan's set of contrary rules, Mrs. Boxley would end up being kept in her state of unalleviated suffering and dementia until taken away by a cardiac arrest or some other dramatic event requiring a more obvious employment of medical technology. Such an approach strikes us as lacking a coherent purpose, namely, the benefit of the patient.

We analyze Mrs. Boxley's case differently. First of all, it does not matter how old she is. She could be 20, 30, 40, or any age up to and beyond her 90s, but she would still not be a candidate for any medical treatment that provided no benefit. Sedation, pain medication, bathing, moistening of the lips—clearly, these would benefit her because she is suffering. Oxygen and antibiotics might also be of help if they alleviated the distress of her pneumonia. All these treatments are aimed at symptoms we believe she is capable of experiencing. But the feeding tube serves no purpose other than keeping her alive to endure more suffering. Therefore, it is futile and should be stopped and replaced by measures undertaken to their maximum powers that provide comfort and dignity.

Misuse of Technology

At the pioneering Seattle Artificial Kidney Center early in the 1960s, patients dying of kidney disease were selected for the newly minted life-saving dialysis treatment by an ethics committee that reviewed criteria including age, gender, marital status, number of dependents, net worth, educational background, occupation, past performance, and future potential. Even letters of recommendation were solicited. This process was adopted by other medical centers around the country. In a short time the anguish experienced by such committees, not to mention that experienced by candidates undergoing the selection process (the majority of whom were necessarily rejected), put pressure on Congress to enact the Medicare End Stage Renal Disease Program in 1972. This amendment provided universal access to treatment at no cost to the patient and under no prescribed limitations. Experts at the time predicted that enrollment in the program would level off by 1992 to 90,000 patients at a cost of between $90 million and $110 million annually.[23]

How prescient were these experts? By 1991 the program was already spending in excess of $5 *billion* annually. Today there are more than 341,000 patients on dialysis and approximately 144,000 recipients of kidney transplants at an annual cost of $35 billion. More than 16,000 kidney transplants were performed in 2008, and almost 80,000 Americans are on waiting lists. And the growth in enrollment shows no sign of leveling off. Indeed, it is predicted to rise to more than $54 billion in 2020 to cover approximately 785,000 patients.[24] As soon as financial barriers were removed, renal dialysis and transplantation began to be offered to patients with conditions that had never been envisioned by the original proponents. Patients with severe diabetes, heart disease, liver disease, and even those in permanent vegetative state started receiving regular and frequent renal dialysis. As one writer commented in the *New England Journal of Medicine:* "The End Stage Renal Disease Program demonstrates the humane impulse that strikes Americans periodically to act on behalf of a vulnerable population. The legislative history of the program suggests that this impulse is driven more by emotions, timing, and the political need to expand benefits than by rational planning."[25]

We have seen this scenario repeated recently with regard to screening mammograms. No sooner did the nonpolitical Preventive Services Task Force recommend against routine mammograms for most women in their 40s based on empirical evidence that until age 50 mammograms showed only a small benefit and considerable harm, then Kathleen Sibelius, secretary of Health and Human Services, responding to public outcry, announced that the report would have no influence on health care policy.[26]

Similarly, intensive care units (ICUs) were developed in the late 1960s to provide a temporary high-technology environment to enable teams of medical providers to rescue patients with acute, serious, life-threatening disease. Patients were expected either to survive and be transferred out of the unit or to die. All this has changed. Today, in our ethics consultations we often discuss patients who have been in the ICU for many months. We are even asked to consult on patients who have inhabited the ICU for more than a year, with no realistic chance of leaving until they die.

Cardiopulmonary resuscitation (CPR) was developed in the 1960s as a rapid emergency procedure to rescue patients with life-threatening cardiac arrest associated with acute myocardial infarction (heart attack). These patients were expected to survive and resume their usual life outside the hospital. Today CPR is attempted on vast numbers of patients who have little chance of surviving even to hospital discharge. Such patients may have terminal cancer or advanced and debilitating failure in several organ systems—lungs, kidneys, heart, liver, bone marrow, and blood—that need continuing support, substitution, or replenishment. In the past, their cardiac arrest, which today is so frantically attacked, would have been considered a welcome event, a "good death," putting a merciful end to their life.

The above examples illustrate how superbly effective advances in medical treatments can become purposeless rituals without reasonable goals. In all of these cases, the intervention was viewed by those first employing it in a far more limited and directed way than has subsequently evolved. One can argue, of course, that there could be many good reasons to expand the applications of an effective technology beyond its original intentions. However, the expansive use of these technologies has often gone unabated and unexamined or simplistically justified on the "life-is-priceless" principle. An example of this attitude is reflected in the glowing publicity in the press of the "feat of surgical wizardry" by surgeons at the Hospital of Philadelphia, who proclaimed the "life-is-priceless" principle to justify their attempted separation of Siamese twin girls with a common heart, which offered one infant no better than 1 percent chance of long-term survival, at a total cost of care that exceeded $1 million. (The child died a year later, never having left the hospital, never having been weaned from a ventilator.)[27] Professor Ronald Dworkin, a scholar of ethics and law responded: "We must face the fact that this is an impossible, even absurd, ideal."[28]

In the first edition of this book we quoted a senior vice president of therapeutics, who justified her pharmaceutical company's $20,000 to $60,000 charge per year for treating a single patient with a single drug, stating: "If there's a scientific way of treating a disease, we have to develop it, and we as a nation have to figure out how to pay for it."[29] Since then, the industry's attitude remains unchanged even while the annual costs of some drugs have risen to the hundreds of thousands of dollars.[30]

Today as we proceed with the complex process of health care reform, we are beginning to see this "unanimous consensus" and "damn-the-torpedoes" attitude being challenged and replaced by calls for research to examine not only the cost but also the effectiveness of treatments in certain clinical circumstances. For example, Dr. Kathy Faber-Langendoen and colleagues, after reviewing the 13-year experience of patients who required mechanical ventilation at the University of Minnesota Bone Marrow Transplant Program, called on physicians to note how abysmal their results were.[31] Of the 191 patients who had to be put on the ventilator, only 6 (3 percent) were alive six months later. None of the patients who required mechanical ventilation within 90 days of the transplant lived more than 100 days, and none of the patients over 40 years of age lived more than a month. And so, after 13 years of employing this invasive treatment, the researchers concluded that mechanical ventilation "is rarely effective in achieving long-term survival in adult BMT [bone marrow transplant] recipients, especially older patients and those early in their transplant course."

Similarly, in another even larger study, two University of Washington intensive care specialists, Gordon Rubenfeld and Steven Crawford, decided to review the medical records of patients who had received bone marrow transplants in perhaps the world's leading center for this procedure. They focused on patients with multiple-organ failure—namely, liver failure, renal failure, and unstable blood pressure—who were put on mechanical ventilators because of inability to maintain normal oxygenation of the blood. To their dismay they discovered that of the 398 patients who met these criteria not a single patient survived to hospital discharge. Their plaintive conclusion portends how difficult they believe it will be to persuade the public to accept the limits of such extreme life-sustaining efforts. "It is difficult to specify limits beyond which treatment should be withheld when there is any chance that a life can be saved. However, if we cannot agree that treating 400 patients with prolonged intensive care without producing a single survivor is beyond such a limit, then it is unlikely we can reach a consensus about limiting care in any clinical situation."[32]

What cannot be forgotten and is particularly tragic is that hundreds of patients were forced to endure the additional pain and suffering and burden of an intervention that resulted in no survival outside the hospital because physicians had never systematically asked the relevant question—Will this intervention make it possible for the patient to survive and leave the hospital or is it futile?—before automatically hooking the patient up to the machine. We also have to recognize the literal brutality of the demand often made by desperate families—"Even if there is only a one in a hundred chance the treatment will work I want you to do it!"—by not losing sight of the denominator. In other words, is it really within the ethical obligation of physicians to subject

100 patients to painful and invasive ICU procedures, including intubation and rib-cracking efforts at CPR, with the faint hope that one patient will survive this torture?

Stephen C. Schoenbaum, a Harvard physician, expressed dismay at the failure of physicians to examine their "bias toward action."[33] Faber-Langendoen, Rubenfeld, and Crawford encountered it, and it propelled the surgeons who inserted Mrs. Boxley's feeding tube.

The Glare of Autonomy

We have already referred to the evolution of the doctor-patient relationship from one that allowed what is now considered excessive paternalism to one that places great emphasis on patient autonomy. This evolution can almost be regarded as a paradigm shift, to adopt an expression used to describe the abrupt changes in the ways scientists historically have viewed the physical world.[34] In the early 1960s, when a group of internists practicing in the United States were asked whether they would inform their patients that they had a grave form of cancer, as many as 90 percent of the physicians expressed reluctance and uncertainty about telling the truth to their patients.[35] A few years later, a similar survey showed exactly the opposite: 90 percent of American physicians studied said they certainly *would* tell the patient the truth.[36] During this period of time—coinciding with the dramatic and much-celebrated social upheavals of the sixties—a remarkable transformation took place in medical teaching and practice.

One of the authors is witness to this vivid change. When he was a medical student in the mid-1950s, a senior physician, who was revered for his compassionate care of patients, gave this advice to all the physicians-in-training after examining on rounds a woman in the last stages of cancer. The frightened woman had asked him directly: "Am I going to die?" He replied kindly, but evasively, "We're all going to die." Later, away from the woman, he counseled us: "Do not tell *her* she has incurable cancer. But make sure someone in the family knows the truth." At the time it was considered the height of clinical wisdom.[37] Today, in the United States, it would be regarded as unthinkable as well as unethical, and even in most cases illegal, not to answer the patient kindly but honestly.

This strong emphasis on "patients' rights" is now a salient and valuable quality in medical decision-making.[38] However, just as physicians abused their kindness in attempting to withhold the truth in the past, sometimes patients abuse the power inherent in their right to make choices about their medical care. Some patients have interpreted their right to control what is done to them by physicians as a right to demand anything they want from physicians. In asserting this right they have created a kind of "glare of autonomy," blinding participants to all other considerations while converting all their desires and dreams into "rights" in a medical context.

In the case of Mrs. Boxley, the glare of autonomy was even more powerful. In the absence of permission from her or from someone empowered to speak on her behalf, the physicians felt blocked from pursuing a course of treatment and care everyone agreed was the most appropriate and humane.

Exhausting the Commons

During medieval and preindustrial times, the central green of a village provided a place for English and other European peasants and yeomen to graze their animals. The commons was a communal resource for the benefit of all, and a sense of restraint initially controlled each family's use of the green. Obviously, if one commoner decided to take advantage of the grazing privilege by adding an extra cow or two, the effect would hardly be noticed. But what if all the neighbors picked up the idea? What if they all increased the number of cows they set out to graze? Eventually all would suffer because the commons would be exhausted. Indeed, over time they did gradually succumb to the temptation to increase their own advantage at the expense of the community at large, and the commons eroded, forcing neighbors to claim and defend sequestered property. Today we often neglect the notion of the commons in our current emphasis on autonomy and individualism. But the concept is relevant to medical resources.[39] In fact, a kind of medical commons exists for all patients. It is not made up merely of material things: institutional space, equipment, supplies and personnel; it consists also of the psyche of caregivers, both loved ones and professionals. These too can become depleted, worn out, exhausted by excessive—and inappropriate—demands.

In the case of Mrs. Boxley, we could see the beginning of serious burnout problems that frequently occur among health providers in high-intensity settings, particularly when they feel they are pursuing measures that have no point. All health care providers—doctors, nurses, social workers—are motivated, trained, and expected to devote their best efforts to either curing or caring for the patients under their responsibility. Every day their efforts are subjected to great physical and emotional pressures. We could sense the wearing down such dedicated, compassionate people feel when they see their efforts consumed and distorted by fruitless demands. And we knew that inevitably, this exhaustion of the commons would affect other patients under their care.

We have also seen an exhaustion of the commons occurring among family members responsible for the care of severely disabled children or severely debilitated adults and elderly individuals.[40] Families will make remarkable sacrifices, rallying to the assistance of one member, as long as the burdens are proportionate to the anticipated outcomes and the benefits to the patient are evident. At times, however, we have seen health providers impose on their own colleagues and on family members an unrealistic patient-centered ethic that fails to recognize the community in which we all draw sustenance. Just as the individual should be respected and valued, so should the community. And so, at times we must say no to futile treatment for no other reason than to prevent the destructive consequences extending to others who are inescapably affected by the treatment of the patient.

Balancing the Claims of Single-Issue Advocates

Nowhere is the balancing of individual needs versus community needs more explicit than in the conflicts that are generated by single-issue advocates. As described in Chapter 1, the members of the Cruzan family were subjected to the aggressive protests of "pro-life" groups seeking to overturn the family's hard-won decision to terminate Nancy Cruzan's treatment. Many such groups have agendas that arise from belief systems they wish to impose on society in general and on the medical profession in particular. During the Reagan and Bush eras, such groups were able to impose a "gag rule" on publicly funded clinics that provided family planning services, including abortion counseling and referral. As in the case of Terri Schiavo, many of these advocacy groups hold a vitalist view of life, condemning any abatement of treatment as long as some biological state, even including permanent unconsciousness, continues. In viewing permanent unconsciousness as another variant of mental disability, they trivialize the needs of patients who really *are* disabled and distract attention from those who really *could* benefit from more resources directed at their needs.

What would these "roving strangers" have done had they been aware of the ethics conference devoted to Mrs. Boxley? It is too easy to imagine a media campaign that ignores the complexity of balancing benefits and burdens by simplistically protesting the horrendous "killing of a poor lonely old woman." Thus, before courts and legislatures bend to such relentless proselytizing, it is important for an enlightened society to make these issues public, to examine them openly and critically. Ultimately, we hope, thoughtful standards will be fashioned that are compatible with both the values of society and the true ends of the medical profession.

Curbing Inappropriate and Covert Abuses

In our ethics consultations we have identified a variety of factors that influence medical treatments. These factors can lead physicians both to curtail and to continue treatments inappropriately. Is the patient old, the disease unattractive, the treatment complicated? Health care providers sometimes find ways to limit their efforts because there are no clear guidelines by which to judge them. Is the patient young, wealthy, important, perhaps even a member of the medical profession? Then no amount of treatment is regarded as too expensive or futile. Does the patient have HIV infection? Physicians and nurses have been reluctant to expose themselves to the risk of HIV no matter how slight.[41] Once again, there are no explicit standards by which to judge the activities of the health care providers. And without some clear set of standards, physicians and patients have no fair and consistent way to examine critically the underlying justification for medical decisions. Thus, we must say no to futile medical treatment as a way of clarifying those treatments that are not futile, those that are obligatory, and those that lie within the realm of patient choice. These steps will serve not only to protect a medical profession fearful of liability, but also to safeguard the interests of patients like Mrs. Boxley.

We began this chapter with the case of Mrs. Boxley, the 92-year-old woman who was transferred to the hospital from a nursing home due to high fever and suspected pneumonia. In a poignant passage from her novel *Death Comes for the Archbishop*, Willa Cather depicts the attitude toward pneumonia taken by elderly people and those who cared for them in an earlier day (the late 1800s). The protagonist, Father Jean Marie Latour, who is dying of pneumonia, accepts both the finality of his life and the inevitability of his own demise. When his young colleague, Bernard, insists, "You should not be discouraged; one does not die from a cold," Cather portrays Father Latour's wise reply: "The old man smiled. 'I shall not die of a cold, my son. I shall die of having lived.'"[42] In modern times, have we lost sight of the fact that death is in store for all of us, that it is the final chapter of life? Because death is never conquered, the goal should be to deal with death honestly, as Cather's protagonist does, evincing as much grace and humility as one can muster.

CHAPTER FOUR

Families Who Say, "Do Everything!"

Helga Wanglie was 85 years old when she had an accident common to all of us, but potentially deadly for elderly people: she tripped on a rug. She tumbled to the floor and broke her hip. During the time it takes for the fracture to heal, patients confined to bed, as Mrs. Wanglie was, can fall prey to developing blood clots, bed sores, and pneumonia. Up to 20 percent of elderly patients who have broken hips die, and many of the survivors never walk again.[1] Many people, though, probably would consider Mrs. Wanglie's outcome—the irreversible unconsciousness of permanent vegetative state—the worst outcome of all.[2] Like Nancy Cruzan before her and Terri Schiavo after her, Helga Wanglie became the object of a nationally publicized lawsuit in 1991 over whether or not to continue life-sustaining treatment in her permanently unconscious condition.

During her hospitalization at Hennepin County Medical Center, in Minneapolis, Mrs. Wanglie developed respiratory failure requiring emergency tracheal intubation and placement on a mechanical ventilator. Despite months of intensive efforts by doctors and technicians, she was never again able to breathe on her own. During these months Mrs. Wanglie remained conscious and aware of her surroundings. She was able to communicate with visiting family members, and she was able to acknowledge when she was in pain or uncomfortable. Yet when asked about her future treatment wishes, she gave ambiguous and inconsistent answers.

She was transferred to a medical facility that specializes in the care of ventilator-dependent patients. There she had a cardiac arrest. Although resuscitated and rushed by ambulance to a nearby acute-care hospital, she never regained consciousness. Faced with clinical signs portending that her unconsciousness would be permanent, a physician asked the patient's husband, son, and daughter to consider withdrawing life-sustaining measures, such as the ventilator. But they refused. Instead, the family arranged to have Mrs. Wanglie moved back to Hennepin County Medical Center. There, after observing her for several weeks, the doctors informed the family of their concurrence that Mrs. Wanglie was in permanent vegetative state and would never recover. They, too, recommended that life-sustaining treatment be withdrawn because it was not benefiting her. But the Wanglie family responded that doctors should not play God, that even suggesting such a step showed moral decay in our civilization, because a miracle could occur.[3]

Mr. Wanglie asserted that life should be maintained as long as possible, no matter what the circumstances, and claimed that his wife, Helga Wanglie, shared this belief. It was never clear, however, whether or not the family's demands to continue life-prolongation represented Mrs. Wanglie's specific wishes or their own. When asked early in his wife's illness, Mr. Wanglie told the medical team that his wife had never discussed her views on life-sustaining treatment. Yet later he asserted, "My wife always stated to me that if anything happened to her so that she could not take care of herself, she didn't want anything done to shorten or prematurely take her life." He claimed to base this view on religious and personal beliefs. "Only God can take life," he said, "and the doctors should not play God."[4]

Over the next several months, the medical team followed the wishes of the patient's family to continue aggressive medical treatment. Mrs. Wanglie was kept on the mechanical ventilator and tube feedings. She was vigorously treated with airway suctioning and antibiotics for recurring pneumonia. Blood tests were performed frequently to facilitate correction of any chemical or fluid imbalances. But because of the irrevocable destruction of her cerebral cortex (demonstrable conclusively by CAT scan) and her multiple medical complications, the medical staff caring for Mrs. Wanglie remained convinced that recovery was impossible and that her life-sustaining ventilator should therefore be discontinued.

At this point, considerations of medical futility were relevant and should, in our view, have been directly addressed. The chance of restoring Mrs. Wanglie to any semblance of consciousness (and the capacity to appreciate any benefit) was nil. In this situation distinct questions arise: Were the physicians caring for Helga Wanglie *ethically obligated* to keep alive a permanently unconscious patient, whose brain was irrevocably destroyed, because the family remained hopeful that "a miracle could occur"? Or were the physicians instead *ethically permitted* to follow their individual conscience in choosing either to withdraw or to continue Mrs. Wanglie's life-sustaining ventilator—guided only by conscience? Or, finally, were the physicians in the Wanglie case ethically bound to act in accordance with professional guidelines and standards of care, and thus as a matter of professional ethics, obligated not to provide futile treatments? We will explore each of these questions in greater detail in Chapter 7.

The hospital's medical director added institutional support to the physicians' appeal to professional standards of care in withdrawing life-sustaining treatment: "All medical consultants agree with [the attending physician's] conclusion that continued use of mechanical ventilation and other forms of life-sustaining treatment are no longer serving the patient's personal medical interest. We do not believe that the hospital is obliged to provide inappropriate medical treatment that cannot advance a patient's personal interest."[5]

Why, then, didn't the health care providers live up to their declared responsibility of withholding "inappropriate medical treatment"? In fact, the clear recognition of medical futility by the medical team was never pursued. Rather, the medical center administration bypassed the physicians and instead consulted their general legal counsel, who chose not to test the issues of medical futility. And rather than following the wishes of the physicians to bring to court the substantive matter—Was Mrs. Wanglie's ventilator futile and were the physicians obligated to provide it?—the Hennepin County Medical Center lawyers chose to engage in a tactical battle with the Wanglie family, a decision that shaped the future course of events.

First, they asked Mr. Wanglie, an attorney himself, to transfer his wife to another hospital more sympathetic with his views, but he refused. The medical center then proposed that if Mr. Wanglie insisted on continuing treatments the physicians regarded as inappropriate, he obtain a court order. Again he refused. The medical center then decided to go to court to remove Mr. Wanglie's decision-making authority.

An interesting sidelight is worth noting. The physicians wanted to test this issue on a patient in whom neither the hospital nor the county had a financial stake in terminating treatment in order to avoid any suggestion of conflict of interest. In fact, they avoided seeking court permission to withdraw treatment on another patient who happened to be in the hospital at the same time in a similar condition—but who relied on Medicaid, publicly funded health insurance for the poor. Medicaid is notorious for low reimbursement rates to physicians and hospitals. The lawyers reasoned that if the doctors or hospital were seen by the media as trying to terminate treatment on a welfare patient, how could they avoid "bad headlines" charging that they were trying to kill patients to save money?

But Mrs. Wanglie's hospital treatment presented no such difficulty. All her costs—approximately $800,000 by the time she died—were fully reimbursed by Medicare and a private supplementary insurance plan. Thus, no one could reasonably claim that the hospital was opposed to Mrs. Wanglie's treatment on grounds of financial self-interest. Yet, unlike the hospital, the Wanglie family had a financial stake in keeping the patient in the hospital. A little known and generally unreported fact in this case was that neither Medicare, the federal health insurance program for the elderly, nor the family's supplementary insurance policy, nor Mrs. Wanglie's pension would cover her costs if she were discharged from the hospital to a nursing home. Medicaid, a public means-tested program, would become available for Mrs. Wanglie's nursing-home care only after she first spent down her personal assets. Unfortunately, this linking of the sacred and the profane is not an unusual experience. Whatever devotion family members might feel for a loved one, whatever their invoking of lofty religious imperatives, any demands for aggressive life-sustaining treatments cannot avoid being influenced by mundane financial matters. Prolonging or curtailing life can have significant consequences on survivors, ranging from the loss of life savings to the termination of monthly disability checks.

In any event, the hospital decided to try to remove Mr. Wanglie from the case. The medical center lawyers asked the court to appoint an independent conservator for Mrs. Wanglie, a person who would have legal authority to decide whether or not the mechanical ventilator keeping her alive was benefiting her. They then hoped for a second hearing on whether or not the hospital was obligated to continue the ventilator if it was deemed nonbeneficial. But Mr. Wanglie intercepted this two-stage strategy by immediately cross-filing, requesting that *he* be appointed his wife's conservator. The court understandably granted his request. Who, the court reasoned, could better represent Helga Wanglie's views and interests than her own husband?

The physicians lacked any direct knowledge of Helga Wanglie's preferences because she did not leave any record of her wishes. Commenting on the Wanglie case, the physician and ethicist Steven Miles has argued that the decision to continue treatment was at odds not only with professional ethics, but also with a growing body of empirical evidence: "A large majority of elderly people prefer not to receive prolonged respirator support for irreversible unconsciousness." He added, "Studies show that an older person's designated family proxy [often] overestimates that person's preference for life-sustaining treatment in a hypothetical coma."[6] Others argued that Mrs. Wanglie's alleged desire for continuous biological existence should not be allowed to compel the medical profession or Mrs. Wanglie's physicians to offer care that is professionally recognized to carry no therapeutic benefit, nor can it compel health insurance companies to pay for medically unnecessary interventions created exclusively by a consumer's demand.[7]

As this case illustrates, the forces leading to the pursuit of futile medical treatment are complex and multifaceted. They can include legal, financial, policy, religious, and other considerations. Nor are they inherently mean-spirited or ill-intentioned. In the Wanglie situation, those who were closest to Mrs. Wanglie—her husband and family—pressed for aggressive treatment. Many families find it difficult to accept the loss of a loved one and want "everything done" as a means of showing their undying love. In fact, many hospital ethics committees share the experience reported by Dr. Edwin H. Cassem, at that time chief of psychiatry and head of the Optimum Care Committee at the Massachusetts General Hospital, that the Wanglie scenario was the most common one to trigger an ethics consultation in that committee's 20-year experience: families insisting that the patient be given treatments physicians regard as futile.[8]

While all this was happening to Helga Wanglie, an even more protracted legal battle was simultaneously unfolding in the state of Florida. Before it was over, the latter conflict would involve more than a dozen trial courts in the longest medical litigation in U.S. history, the state and federal government, even the president of the United States of America—all under the glare of national and international media. The patient was the 27-year-old Terri Schiavo.

Terri Schiavo had a cardiac arrest early one February morning in 1990, possibly as a result of a potassium deficiency secondary to an eating disorder. Firefighters and paramedics responded to her husband's 911 call and managed to restart her heart, but she never regained consciousness. At first, her devoted husband (Michael Schiavo) and her mother and father (Robert and Mary Schindler) pursued every effort to keep her alive and restore her to consciousness, including arranging speech and occupational therapy, even flying her to the University of California, San Francisco, for a failed experimental implantation of a brain stimulator. However, by 1993, after coming to terms with the physicians' judgments that so much of her higher brain function was irreversibly lost that there was no longer any hope for his wife's recovery, Michael Schiavo, who was the patient's legal guardian (as well as a nurse), requested that a Do Not Resuscitate Order be entered into Terri Schiavo's nursing home record.

At this point, Terri Schiavo's parents and husband parted ways and became locked in a vitriolic and public combat in the courts and in the media.[9] Five years later (in 1998) Mr. Schiavo filed a petition in court to remove her feeding tube. He stated that his wife told him and relatives on several occasions that she would not want to have her life artificially prolonged.[10] Although lower courts generally sided with Mr. Schiavo, and the feeding tube was eventually removed, the case quickly became a rallying point for conservative religious groups. By October, 2004, the Florida legislature had become involved, passing a one-time-only law that reversed a series of lower court rulings and empowered Florida's governor, Jeb Bush, to order the feeding of Mrs. Schiavo through a tube. Mr. Schiavo appealed to the Florida Supreme Court, which found the law unconstitutional and a violation of the separation of church and state.[11] Even Pope John Paul II became involved when he issued an allocution to the clergy (which Robert and Mary Schindler, who are Roman Catholic, promptly submitted to the court) that it is wrong in principle to withhold food and water from people in a persistent vegetative state.[12]

Like the Helga Wanglie case, the Terri Schiavo case brought forth repeated testimony from experienced neurologists that the patient was permanently unconscious and would never be aware of, much less benefit from, being kept biologically alive. In other words, the life-sustaining efforts produced biological effects but were futile because the patient would never have the capacity to appreciate those effects as a benefit. In the final analysis, though, the judgment of the court was based not on the uselessness of the available treatments, but on what the patient's wishes would be under the circumstances. The question courts focused on and debated was: What would this young woman in a permanent vegetative state—a condition she almost certainly never heard of nor even imagined—have wanted? The answer the court was seeking required a leap of imagination and testimony from witnesses that would not have met the standards for "clear and convincing evidence" in other states.[13] Yet their testimony persuaded the Florida court that she had made "reliable oral declarations that she would have wanted the feeding tube removed." The feeding tube was removed, and Terri Schiavo died in a hospice facility on March 31, 2005. An autopsy showed the brain to be reduced to half normal weight with extensive damage to all regions, which, in the words of the chief medical examiner, was "irreversible, and no amount of therapy or treatment would have regenerated the massive loss of neurons." In short, whatever her wishes, all efforts to restore Terri Schiavo to consciousness were futile.

Why Do Families and Loved Ones Say, "Do Everything!"?

Why do families and loved ones make such demands, pleading for treatments that are against all reason? How should physicians and other health professionals respond to such demands?

In a personal anecdote, the medical ethicist Norman Daniels provides insight into the universality of the Wanglie phenomenon: the conflicted emotional state that assails families who want "everything done," including medical treatments that are prolonged beyond the point of usefulness. He recounted how his aged great-aunt became seriously ill and was rushed to an intensive-care hospital, where exhaustive efforts were made to extend her life. The woman's daughter (Professor Daniels's cousin) sought to reassure him: "The doctors are doing everything to save her." But when Daniels suggested that "perhaps it was time to let her die peacefully," he was rebuked: "It's my mother—I can't do that." Daniels then asked his cousin whether she would want her own daughter to treat her some day the way she was treating her mother. "God forbid," she exclaimed. "When my time comes, I just want to go."[14]

The striking feature about this exchange is how it exposes the contrast between what we want for ourselves and what we demand, or feel obligated to provide, for those we love. Is this why Mr. Wanglie found it so difficult to agree to stop medical treatments that were doing his wife no good? Did the decision uncover deep feelings of guilt or animosity in relation to his wife? Did he perceive the life-extending treatments to be a way of proving his "undying" love, demanding them in order to meet his obligation as a good and faithful husband? Was the idea of allowing Mrs. Wanglie to die tainted by a sense that withdrawing life-prolonging treatment would signify that she was unworthy of respect and dignity? Had the treatments become transformed into a symbolic ritual? Had they been diverted into a means of benefiting Mr. Wanglie, rather than his wife, a way of postponing his own inevitable loss? Similar questions could be asked about the Schindlers (Terri Schiavo's parents). What could be more painful than losing an only child? What associations and symbolic meanings did withdrawal of nutrition and hydration have for Ms. Schiavo's parents, given the context of their daughter's eating disorder, which likely led to her cardiac arrest? To what extent did feelings of guilt and responsibility, need for control, and denial and unwillingness to face death, feed the parents' drive to continue the tube feedings? While the details are unique for every case, these stories share a common thread: family members demanding "heroic" medical measures to demonstrate love, show concern and compassion, and deny what is really going on in a situation.

Daniels's story reveals how our love for another person can cause us to demand more for that person than we would demand (or even permit) for ourselves. Boundless love suggests that there can be no limits to what we owe to the object of our love. Yet, making extraordinary (and useless) efforts as an expression of love has an empty ring to it when those efforts do not benefit the object of love. If Mr. Wanglie were intent on proving his love for his wife, he chose ways that did not benefit *her*. She was beyond all comprehension. We can perhaps understand the depth of his feelings; but must we require that the doctors, nurses, and other health-care providers—indeed, society at large—participate in gestures that do not serve the best interests of the patient, his wife?

It is helpful to contrast our demands for loved ones not only with our desires for ourselves but also with our perceived obligations to other people—strangers. Philosophers observe that we tend to feel we owe more to those with whom we are intimate than we owe to complete strangers. The special obligations that flow from personal relationships are not only stronger in degree but different in kind. Friends and family members may feel an unlimited obligation to provide nurturing, personal time, life savings, even life itself. Indeed, lovers sometimes do take their own lives rather than be without their loved ones—though this serves no useful purpose to the loved one. What has happened, of course, is that the person one loves may have become such a central part of a person's life that the loss of that person is tantamount to losing one's *self*. Perhaps underneath Mr. Wanglie's demands for continued treatment was the question he could not face: If I am no longer her husband, who am I?

And so, regardless of whether we owe unlimited expressions of love to spouses, siblings, children, and parents, it is not surprising that we *feel* that we do. Ordinarily, going out of our way to help those we love strengthens and reinforces the bonds of our relationships. In the medical setting, however, when treatment becomes futile, "doing everything" can become a cruel parody. It is not that the impulse to do everything possible is itself wrongheaded; rather we need to rethink what it means to do our utmost when a loved one is hopelessly ill and dying. In Mrs. Wanglie's case, for example, Mr. Wanglie would have done the utmost for his wife by allowing her to die with as much kindness and dignity as possible, free of useless life-sustaining machinery. Likewise, after years of devotedly seeking a cure, Michael Schiavo finally chose to acknowledge the fact that his wife would not recover. He expressed his love for her by allowing her final days to be dignified and free of invasive tubes and medical procedures from which she could not appreciate any benefit.

What about the health professionals? Rather than unthinkingly following Mr. Wanglie's demands, the health-care providers would have better lived up to their professional obligations to Mrs. Wanglie by supporting actions that, when the alternatives became futile, allowed her to become part of a cherished past as a beloved person rather than as a permanent vegetative "state."

How Should Physicians Respond to Demands for Futile Treatment?

John Paris, a priest, and Frank E. Reardon, a philosopher, issue the challenge very bluntly: "How do we respond to families and physicians who seek refuge from unwanted painful reality in futile end-stage gestures?"[15] Some find the answer all too easy: Patients and families are entitled to full decision-making authority, including even irrational choices, as protection against "the medical profession's intent and power to maintain its paternalistic authority."[16] But

Paris and Reardon have little patience with that notion: "With an approach that places near control in the hands of the patient, no moral legitimacy is given to a physician's refusal of requested treatment. The physician is reduced from moral agent—one with professional responsibilities and limits on what may legitimately be done—and transformed into an extension of the patients' (or families') whim, fantasy or unrealizable hopes and desires. Such a relationship not only distorts the physician's role, it destroys the very autonomy it was designed to enhance."[17]

We agree. Do we really want physicians to be forced to include "whim, fantasy, or unrealizable hopes and desires" in their therapeutic armamentarium? Without "at least a modicum of potential benefit, as seen from the medical perspective," ethicists Allan Brett and Laurence B. McCullough argue, "the whole raison d'être of the physician-patient interaction disappears."[18]

Sometimes, of course, it seems easier to submit to unreasonable demands than to challenge them. But what are patients (or more often their families) really asking from physicians?[19]

In a poignant letter to the editor of the *New York Times*, Janet Rivkin Zuckerman complained that physicians who unquestioningly pursue futile treatments either out of misguided duty or in response to families' demands demonstrate a distressing poverty of imagination: "Isn't it possible that if physicians were more highly developed and educated in doctor-patient relations—that is, in empathy, understanding and communication—it would offset their driving need always to *do* something?"[20] In other words, it struck Ms. Zuckerman that in looking for empathy, understanding, and communication, patients and families want physicians not to become reflexive automatons. Yes, patients and families want their physicians to be skillful and knowledgeable masters of the science and technology of medicine. But they also want their physicians to be wise counselors whose understanding embraces not only their patient's biology but also the patient's humanity.

Underlying many of the demands to "do everything" is the fear of abandonment. Does the doctor consider me (or my loved one) no longer worthy of her attention? There are many indirect ways these fears may be expressed by the patient or by the patient's loved ones. For example, Robert M. Veatch and Carol Mason Spicer, two Kennedy Institute ethicists, describe a 36-year-old man admitted to the hospital with symptoms of advanced AIDS: "He was placed on a ventilator and became mentally incompetent. The clinicians concluded that further aggressive care would be futile, but the patient's lover intervened, saying that he and the patient had discussed these matters openly and that the patient had asked that everything be done. He was quoted as saying, 'Don't let them give up on me.' "[21] Veatch and Spicer draw the conclusion from this heart-rending plea that by "everything" the patient meant all the *life-prolonging* procedures in the medical arsenal, including presumably attempted CPR, mechanical ventilation, renal dialysis, major surgery, or whatever else might conceivably be of use to keep the man's body alive.

But we regard this as a simplistic interpretation of what patients and loved ones are asking for, and what medicine can rightly offer. We therefore draw a far different conclusion in this case. For us, the patient's cry poignantly reveals what has become lost in medical practice and what is missing in the futility debate: the bedside art of spending time with the patient, listening, and providing patients the opportunity to express themselves and know they are being acknowledged and cared for. If medical decision-making at the end of life is nothing more than a tug of war limited to whether to "pull the plug" or "pound on the chest," then the patient who is not offered life-prolonging treatment might reasonably wonder: Do the doctors deem me unworthy of their time and concern? Am I no longer of value? Am I being discarded? Understandably, the patient or the patient's loved ones might respond with a desperate plea to "do everything."

Yet for us, "doing everything and "not giving up" on the patient is not literally a request for the physician to use every technology available. Instead, it speaks to the patient's vulnerability and need for—in addition to optimal comfort care—human connection and support. It is a plea for others to remain present with the patient, express loyalty, impart meaning, and ultimately contribute dignity to the patient's final chapter of life. In our experience, dying patients do not want their last days to be spent bound and mummified in machines and tubes, nor subjected to painful and disabling procedures. Instead, decoding the request for "everything possible," reveals that patients (and families), who admittedly may be in denial and unprepared to let go, are seeking human love, recognition, and support. Surely there are better ways of providing what they are seeking than inflicting futile medical treatments.

Too often the futility debate degenerates into an intractable conflict between physician and patient (or surrogate or family member) over who decides whether or not a particular life-saving treatment should be attempted. Those who argue on behalf of physician-determined futility will emphasize the limits of the medical profession's obligations to provide inappropriate treatments. In rebuttal, those on the opposing side who proclaim the unlimited rights of patients to choose any treatments, even irrational treatments, will express a number of concerns, in particular that granting physicians the power to withhold treatment on the grounds of medical futility will reverse recent gains in patients' rights against medical paternalism. They also will warn that physicians could use futility as an excuse to arbitrarily abandon patients in covert acts of rationing or for other unethical reasons. Sadly, this debate distracts the medical team from concentrating their efforts on all the possibilities of comfort care it can provide to dying patients in the final days and hours of life.

Beyond Futility to an Ethic of Care

In this narrow debate we, together with Dr. Kathy Faber-Langendoen, have argued that a crucial element is overlooked, both at the bedside and in public commentary. The physician has an ethical duty to redirect efforts from life-prolonging treatments toward the aggressive pursuit of treatments that maximize comfort and dignity for the patient and for the grieving family.[22]

An *ethic of care* has a long-standing and prominent place in the history of medicine,[23] summarized nicely in the fifteenth-century French adage, "to cure sometimes, to relieve often, to comfort always." Unfortunately, the historical development of scientific medicine and the rising status of physicians have sometimes placed physicians at odds with such activities as expressing empathy and care. Little in their training today is devoted to improving their abilities of engagement and identification with others. As one of us (NSJ) has argued elsewhere, reemphasizing an ethic of care in medicine may lead to "positive changes in bioethical education, including placing greater emphasis on health care providers' communication skills and emotional sensitivity."[24]

We find an ethic of care most clearly articulated in the nursing literature, where it is defined as a commitment to protecting and enhancing the patient's dignity.[25] Caring goes beyond good intentions or simple kindness and includes psychological, philosophic or religious, and physical components, taking into consideration the patient's social context and specific goals. And although "caring" is used in different ways, we use this term to refer specifically to emotional connections between persons that include affective, cognitive, and volitional dimensions. All three aspects are important. An *affective* dimension is key to caring because unless one actually "feels with" the person, pleased and relieved when the person is doing well, worried or anxious when the person is not, one does not really care. A *cognitive* component is essential because merely feeling concerned is not sufficient; one must also have knowledge and understanding of the other person's needs, welfare, and circumstances. Finally, a *volitional* dimension is necessary to caring because to care means not only to want what is good for another, but to act in bringing this about.[26]

The concept of palliative care, which emphasizes the relief of symptoms and the easing of pain, is becoming increasingly accepted by physicians and used in acute-care hospitals, in designated palliative care units, and in institutional and home-based hospice programs. As Jecker and Self note, historically, it was American nursing, not medicine, that was linked with care-giving activities in the domestic sphere: mothers, daughters, and sisters nursed their families at home, sometimes aided by female neighbors who called themselves "professed" or "born" nurses and had previous experience caring for their own families.[27] By contrast, American physicians "achieved professional status and identity by fashioning a separate sphere. Given the association between caring and 'women's work', physicians had little incentive to identify their own professional function as caring."[28] Yet although caregiving remains largely the domain of nurses (and women), physicians who care *about* patients engage emotionally with the patient. In other words, they show an attitude, feeling, or state of mind directed toward the patient and the patient's situation. As Jecker and Self note, caring about "requires keeping the patient's best interest in the forefront of mind and heart."[29]

The call to emphasize an ethic of care when disease can no longer be cured or controlled requires strengthening collaborative efforts among health care professionals. Physicians and nurses have much to learn from one another, as well as from experts in hospice care and those conducting research into ways to improve palliative care.[30] For example, physicians owe to hospice nurses the discovery that treatments aimed at keeping dying patients well hydrated with intravenous fluids often *add* to patient discomfort by worsening respiratory secretions and dyspnea.[31] And contrary to popular perceptions of neglect, if patients are allowed to die without tubes in their veins and gut, forcing foods and fluids into their bodies, they may very well get to enjoy the sedative and euphoric benefits of metabolic acidosis.[32]

Changing perceptions about the physician's role as caregiver will require active educational efforts by health professionals. Health professionals should also be advocates for creating institutional facilities that permit patients the option of dying in the privacy and presence of loved ones and friends, rather than in the far more usual (and impersonal) setting of ICUs, surrounded by the instruments of high technology and bustling and intrusive hospital providers. Making these alternatives available—giving patients and families these choices—will be achieved, we hope, by better reimbursement and support for home-based and hospice services.

While an ethic of care is sometimes seen as coming into force only when a cure can no longer be expected, it is fitting that the French dictum was to comfort *always*. A view of medicine that sees care and cure as diametrically opposed values ill-serves patients who need compassion and relief of troubling symptoms even in the midst of potentially curative therapy. However, when medical intervention is futile in achieving the goals of curing or ameliorating disease, the comfort of the patient rises to the fore as the primary attainable goal. As it assumes this primacy, all medical interventions can be critically examined to see if they contribute to the patient's comfort; those that do not aid the patient's comfort ought to be discarded.

Finally, better caring for patients when medical treatment is futile calls for public education and improved communication between health professionals and patients. As Dr. Timothy Quill noted, "Sharing feelings . . . with an empathic listener can be the first step toward healing. At [the very] least, isolation is taken out of the doubt and despair."[33] Note Quill's emphasis on healing, which takes as its object the person, not a biological organism or (worse) a body part or organ system. Sitting down and talking with the patient, and thereby recognizing the patient as a person, helps to give voice to the patient's concerns and fears, validate the patient's feelings, educate the patient about what to expect, and humanize the dying process for both the health professional and the patient. Moreover, sensitive exploration of the patient's or the family's request for a futile treatment will often yield avenues of help that were previously unanticipated and that are acceptable to all parties. Rather than assuming a confrontational stance, it is worth taking time to explore the patient's and/or the family's feelings. Fears of abandonment, for example, can be addressed by turning the attention of the family and the medical team attention to working intensively with a dying patient to minimize pain and suffering, address psychosocial and spiritual issues, and prepare for death. And denial of death can be addressed through a counseling process that helps the patient or the family to face and find meaning in the dying process. Although "merely sitting down and getting to know" the patient is derided by some physicians as "soft" medicine, or even eliminated from the physician's role altogether and delegated to other health professionals (social workers and nurses), responsible and humane medicine cannot occur without it. It is only through exploration of the latent content of requests for futile interventions that physicians can achieve medicine's goal of healing the patient.

All too often, patients demand futile treatments because of the symbolic message such treatment conveys: that the medical team is displaying the utmost concern for the patient by using the most modern, invasive technologies. When such aggressive approaches are not used, patients and families express feelings of abandonment; families (and others) use words such as "starvation" and "neglect" to describe patients who are not connected to intravenous lines, gastrostomy tubes, or ventilators. We wish to emphasize that futile interventions are poor ways of promoting caring and compassion. Futile treatments make a mockery of caring by substituting technology for human communication and touch.

Medicine, like all human endeavors, has its own inevitable limits. While these limits may shift with advances in technology and science, it is deceptive to act as though medicine can conquer all disease, or even death itself. Nor is it sufficient merely to refrain from offering or employing futile interventions that do not work. Rather, we urge that the discussion of futility move beyond definitional debates to promote a positive ethic of care, including research and educational efforts into the care of patients when those inevitable limits are reached. Overlooked in the perspective limited to attempting life-prolonging treatments is a whole set of obligations that involve not only aggressive attacks on the dying process but also the physician's duty to enhance the patient's comfort and dignity maximally during the last days of life, including aggressively working to alleviate pain and suffering.

Again, we must emphasize that patients and families who "demand everything" are not entitled to demand miracles of the medical profession. And again we acknowledge that medicine—through marketing and other strategies of self-promotion—is sometimes a shameful participant in fostering miraculous expectations among the lay public.[34] But physicians are not and never were obligated to treat in expectation of a miracle. We would even press the argument further: Attempting futile treatments is irresponsible and should be condemned by the profession.

There are innumerable goals that persons strive for in the course of living and dying. Happiness, religious peace, reconciliation with estranged family, a sense of having fought to the death with honor—these are all goals that, although laudable and brought into sharp focus by disease, are beyond the reach of medicine. Ill health and the prospect of one's death confront the individual with many perplexing problems, only some of which can be addressed by physicians' remedies. While physicians are fundamentally obligated to comfort patients, it is arrogant to pretend that physicians are equipped to fulfill every conceivable desire.[35]

How Should Physicians Respond to Families Who Say, "Do Everything!"?

The physicians caring for Helga Wanglie and Terri Schiavo expended great time, care, and compassion in trying to persuade family members to allow them to discontinue what all the health care providers concluded was inappropriate medical treatment that did not serve to benefit these two individuals. Thus in fairness to the doctors, nothing short of a declaration of medical futility, supported by institutional and societal values, would have sufficed. In many other situations, however, we have discovered that families' demands are not so intractable if the subtext of their demands are understood and addressed. In our experience, physicians and families welcome discussions that involve not only the negative act of withholding and withdrawing life-sustaining treatment but also the positive act of enhancing the last remaining days of life. These discussions should neither be confined to obtaining a simple yes or no about a particular procedure nor be typified by the physician's turning all care over to the nursing staff. Rather, such plans should provide strategies for maximizing comfort and dignity in the waning hours and days of life within the context of all that surrounds that patient, including family and friends.

In this regard, physicians and nurses are morally obligated to use narcotics, sedatives, tranquilizers, and other palliative measures with the same professional skill they apply to any other treatment efforts. Continuing to draw blood, insert feeding tubes, or surround the patient with monitors and other invasive technologies should be avoided unless they clearly contribute to the patient's well-being.[36] If physicians, as a profession, are granted the responsibility to make determinations of medical futility, they are all the more obligated to act according to an ethic of care. In particular, this will require better collaborative, interdisciplinary efforts among all health care professionals. At present, physicians and nurses, despite generations of collaborative efforts on behalf of patients, too often exist in separate professional and social worlds. They have much to gain from breaking down the barriers that separate them— as well as from breaking down barriers between them and experts from hospice and others who are conducting research into ways to improve palliative care.

We hope that in the future, patients and providers who want "everything done" will direct their efforts and emotional energies not to useless treatments that serve only to magnify suffering and threaten human dignity but to treatments that work to the maximum benefit of the patient.[37] Saying no to futile treatment does not mean saying no to caring for the patient; rather, it means transferring aggressive efforts away from life *prolongation* and toward life *enhancement* in the waning hours and days of existence. Ideally, "doing everything" means optimizing the potential for a good life,[38] and then permitting that most important coda to a good life—a "good death."[39]

CHAPTER FIVE

Futility and Rationing

Juanita was an eight-year-old Mexican girl who had acute lymphocytic leuke-mia. Her mother would transport her across the border to a university medical center in the United States whenever her daughter began to lose weight and become severely weak. The university hospital doctors who made the original diagnosis and prescribed the chemotherapy treated her even though they knew she was not a U.S. citizen and could not afford to pay. Each time they advised her mother to continue follow-up treatment in Mexico. Instead, every few months the mother brought the girl to them, each time with her disease in an advanced stage of relapse. The woman claimed she was unable to obtain the necessary treatment in her own country.

This time the hematologists faced a situation that was particularly grim. The disease was now resistant to the available chemotherapy drugs, and any more radical treatment, such as total body radiation and bone marrow trans-plantation, was hazardous, expensive, and not very promising. The mother—who had relentlessly pursued what she regarded as the best treatment in the United States—pleaded with the doctors to do everything possible to save her daughter's life. The doctors were in a quandary. Because they knew the mother and daughter from previous encounters, they had begun to feel a special relationship with them. And, of course, they wanted to save Juanita's life if they could.

What should they do? It was clear at this point that even the most aggressive treatments had an exceedingly small chance of saving Juanita's life. But were the chances so vanishingly small as to consider them futile? While sorting that out among themselves, they could not ignore a further consideration. She was not a citizen of the United States and thus not legally entitled to treatment (under Medicaid). The question therefore arose whether or not Juanita was *ethically* entitled to treatment: Was it fair for U.S. physicians to offer a noncitizen scarce and expensive resources, resources that were paid for by U.S. taxpayers as part of a public insurance program (Medicaid)? The question of how to ethically distribute scarce resources is what philosophers call the problem of distributive justice.

In a just society, one seeks to achieve a fair distribution of benefits and burdens. In the case of Juanita, the benefits were obviously medical treatments that could save her life. But neither she nor anyone in her family had participated in sharing the burdens, such as taxes, that go to pay for hospital care. (Ironically, of course, being poor, they probably would not have had sufficient income to pay U.S. taxes in comparison with the welfare support they received. But still, they would have been exposed to all the obligations of citizenship, including tax burdens.)

In this example, the question of whether or not to provide Juanita a bone marrow transplant raises issues of both rationing and futility. With respect to *rationing,* one concern is the *relatively* low likelihood and quality of medical benefit. That is, relative to other patients who might receive this treatment, Juanita's quality and likelihood of benefit was comparatively poor. The basis for *futility* also involves evaluating the potential benefits of treatment, but only with regard to the *individual patient* and not relative to any other patients. If the likelihood or quality of benefit Juanita herself would receive from the transplant fails to approach a threshold considered minimal, then the transplant can be withheld on the basis of medical futility.

The Different Connotations of Rationing and Futility

The doctors struggled mightily with the decision about what to do for Juanita. They worried about their objectivity in evaluating her condition and treatment prospects. Were they unconsciously underestimating the chances of success in attempting aggressive and expensive bone marrow transplantation because Juanita's mother was not a tax-paying American citizen legally entitled to medical benefits? In other words, were they *inappropriately invoking medical futility*? Or were they so emotionally bonded to the child that they could not accept that she was not legally qualified for this limited and highly expensive medical procedure, which almost certainly would not help her anyway? Were they thereby *inappropriately invoking rationing*? What lay at the root of their struggle?

One possible explanation lies in the historical contexts and connotations we commonly associate with rationing. Acknowledging the need to ration violates the cherished ideal that no member of society should be considered less worthy and less desirable than any other. Because rationing involves weighing the claims of different persons, it is by its very nature discriminatory. Futility, by contrast, is concerned with the benefits treatment can produce for only a single patient. It does not make comparisons between patients. And yet, a paradox arises. When physicians are confronted with a patient who succumbed to an illness despite their best efforts, when in fact the *treatment* failed, physicians often report that "the *patient* failed the treatment."

Perhaps underlying the physicians' discomfort was the notion that there is something sinister in the concept of rationing. Some people simplistically impute spiraling medical costs to singular malign influences—too many lawyers, too greedy doctors, too powerful insurance companies. They hold that resource and financial restrictions could be done away with if only people were more generous, more pure of heart. If only society, they argue, were capable of abolishing the forces of self-interest, rationing could be done away with altogether. Futility arouses quite different concerns. It suggests that there simply is nothing anyone can do—as though the doctor is merely reporting an objective fact, rather than making a value-laden judgment. Futility does not suggest a shortage of resources or failure of generosity, only a limit to human capacity.

The Reasons for Greater Attention to Futility and Rationing

Why are we talking about rationing and futility at all? Why have these twin topics gained such prominence in recent years? A number of factors are no doubt responsible.

The Rise in Health Care Costs

To begin with, increasing health care costs represent a growing source of public and professional concern. The price of health care has risen at a faster rate than other consumer prices. As noted in Chapter 3, expenditures on health care now amount to about $2.5 trillion a year and roughly $6,600 spending per person.[1]

Comparing current figures with those of prior years helps to convey their significance. In 1960, for example, national health care expenditures represented just 5.3 percent of the gross national product (now called gross domestic product), and in 1970, 7.4 percent; by 1985, that figure had jumped to 10.7 percent, and now it is more than 17 percent. These increased health care expenditures cannot be explained by economic growth and gains in productivity alone, but have required the transfer of resources from other areas of the economy.[2] These economic facts lead many to call for measures to "cap" health care spending. One direct response to this call for limits is increased attention to rationing health care. Undoubtedly, the debate over medical futility represents an *indirect* response to the same economic circumstances. But acknowledgment of this fact should not invalidate the search for a definition of medical futility. After all, the most attractive method of containing health care costs would be to trim the fat out of the system.[3] Because futile treatments are, by definition, of no benefit, they should be the first to go.

On the other hand, under conditions of scarcity, even *beneficial* medical treatments may be denied. When even beneficial resources are scarce, the question is not whether to ration, but how to ration. Will it be done in an explicit fashion? Or will de facto rationing instead proceed in a covert and unsystematic manner? In organ transplantation, for example, potential recipients greatly outnumber donors, and rationing is clearly needed. Even where no significant shortage exists in the resources required to produce medical services, money to pay for medical care is itself limited. For example, whether at 12 percent, 17 percent, or 25 percent, an upper limit on the amount of gross domestic product devoted to health care inevitably will occur. This is because continued increases in health care spending divert public funds from other social goods, such as education, transportation, law enforcement, and the environment. Thus, medical treatments are evaluated, compared, and rationed on the basis of cost as well as benefit.

The Development of High-Technology Medicine

A second reason that the topics of futility and rationing command greater attention of late has to do with medical success and the development of high-technology medicine. By "high technology," we mean apparatus and procedures based on modern sciences, as opposed to simpler healing arts; new, as opposed to long-accepted methods; scientifically complex, as distinct from commonsense approaches; costly, rather than inexpensive treatments; and limited, rather than widespread, expertise in using a particular technique.[4]

The historically recent availability of new, effective medical technologies brings to the fore issues of both futility and rationing. Early in the development of a new technology, there will be the question of establishing whether it is effective. After a new procedure has established its effectiveness, it will often present issues of justice in the distribution of limited resources. This is due, in part, to the developer's search for ways to maximize profit and recover the high cost associated with the technology's research, development, and delivery. The developer's marketing strategy will often involve promoting new applications for the technology. Each new technology inevitably competes with others for hospital space, insurance coverage, and trained personnel. In the beginning, the number of health professionals trained to apply a new technique in the clinical setting may be limited. As more health care providers are trained, they inevitably seek out more patients on whom to apply their new medical advance.

This insidious expansion beyond the original objective could be considered the medical version of what the military calls "mission creep." When a new technology appears on the scene, it almost always is rationed, at first because it is limited; later, as it becomes more widespread, it is rationed because its expanded application is found to be costly and only marginally beneficial for certain groups of patients. Such rationing rarely takes place explicitly and according to publicly stated criteria; it is more often done implicitly and without acknowledgment and deliberation.

After a new technology becomes more widely available, the ethical problems it raises may turn from that of justly distributing a scarce medical resource to that of limiting its inappropriate use. Enthrallment with new techniques, together with the prestige sometimes associated with their use or the financial remuneration they command, may encourage excessive use, thereby exacerbating the ethical problem of medical futility. In medicine this is a recurrent story: initially a new technique is employed for a limited group of patients who can be shown clearly to benefit. Soon, however, the "indications" for the technique expand. More patients who can benefit only marginally "qualify" for the treatment. (This is sardonically referred to as the "hammer and nail" phenomenon: to the hammer, every problem is a nail.)

For example, renal dialysis—which was a dramatic technology originally developed to provide life support for patients until they recovered from temporary kidney failure—now is far more often used to keep alive patients whose kidney failure is permanent. As we noted in Chapter 3, this expansion of the technology was explicitly (and impulsively) sanctioned by society when Congress, moved by emotional hearings featuring patients hooked up to dialysis machines, enacted the End Stage Kidney Disease funding program, which guaranteed funding to cover treatment for all patients in need. What society did *not* sanction or even envision are the many uses of renal dialysis that take place today, including keeping alive unconscious patients in a permanent vegetative state, who will never perceive any benefit, and advanced metastatic cancer patients, who will never be well enough to leave the hospital.

Another medical intervention, tube feeding—originally applied to patients who could not take food by mouth but were otherwise capable of benefiting from their existence—was expanded to include even permanently unconscious patients. In two states, New York and Missouri, courts specifically held that family members and others close to the patient have no authority to refuse this treatment unless the patient has signed a health care proxy—which only a small fraction of patients ever had the foresight to execute.

Another good example of technology with expanding indications is cardiopulmonary resuscitation (CPR). Again, this procedure originally was developed for patients with acute transient and largely reversible medical conditions, such as sudden cardiac arrest secondary to myocardial infarction (heart attack). Today, though, CPR is attempted on any number of patients who experience a cardiac arrest, regardless of their underlying disease or quality of life.[5]

This policy of "presumed demand" for CPR prompted bioethicists Tom Tomlinson (a philosopher) and Howard Brody (a physician) to ask why attempted CPR was undertaken indiscriminately, rather than viewed like any other treatment.[6] According to their view (and ours), any decision to withhold attempted CPR on grounds of medical futility falls within the physician's professional responsibility and expertise. As with any other treatment, they argue, attempted CPR should be offered only if it can benefit the patient.

In contrast to rationing, the main thrust of this appeal is not that the re-sources or staff available to serve a group of patients are limited, but rather that treatment is not medically beneficial for an individual patient. Naturally, skeptics may wonder, "Is futility invoked to disguise rationing? Would the issue of futility be raised in the absence of competition for limiting resources?"

The Aging of Society

A third element directing greater focus on futility and rationing is the aging of society. Although the population of most developed countries has been aging since 1800, the pace of aging has accelerated greatly in recent years. Since 1900, for example, the United States has witnessed an eightfold increase in the number of people over the age of 65. Those over the age of 85, the fastest-growing age group in the country, are 21 times as numerous as in 1900. The elderly are also the heaviest users of health services. Persons 65 and over represent approximately 12 percent of the U.S. population but account for about one-third of the nation's total personal health care expenditures, exclusive of research costs.

The phenomenon of an aging society has led some to question public funding of life-extending health care in old age. Allan Meltzer, an economist at Carnegie Mellon University, notes that about 2 percent of the entire gross domestic product goes to Medicare payments for people who are within six months of dying. He then adds bluntly, "And I think that is a waste."[7] According to ethicist Daniel Callahan, even if life-extending medical care were un-limited, elderly people themselves would be wise to settle for the achievement of a limited natural lifespan.[8] The suggestion is not that public investments in life-extending therapies for older individuals produce no medical benefit; rather, these treatments are futile in a broad sense: death in old age is inevi-table, and an acceptance of limits is therefore fitting.

This broader sense of futility suggested by Meltzer and Callahan should not be confused with our own definition. Callahan's definition is not based on medical criteria, such as the poor likelihood of achieving medical benefits for older patients or the low quality of medical benefits in older age groups. In-deed, such an approach would be difficult to sustain, as evidence is mounting that there is no significant correlation between age and mortality or morbidity outcomes associated with various interventions, including survival after CPR for in-hospital cardiac arrests and coronary arteriography, liver and kidney transplantation and other surgeries, chemotherapy, and dialysis.[9] Rather than basing his concept of futility on medical criteria, Callahan uses a strictly age-based approach, drawing a line at an upper age range. By contrast, we define futility in terms of medical outcomes and perceive no necessary correlation between the futility of an intervention and the age of a patient.

Despite the lack of evidence showing that older individuals consistently experience poorer medical outcomes, elderly people recently have become a target for denial of care based on rationing as well as futility. The appeal of age-based rationing is due in part to the fact that the ranks of older Americans are swelling and the cost of care for elderly people is disproportionately high. While not all agree that rationing health care based on age is ethically or philosophically sound, several arguments are advanced in support of such a proposal. Productivity arguments hold that the goal of maximizing life-years saved, or costs saved, or contributions to the public good, can best be achieved by limiting the health care to elderly people. Other arguments claim that if individuals were to view their lives as a whole, rather than at a particular moment in time, their considered preferences would be to distribute more medical resources to earlier, rather than later, years.[10]

Limits on Patient Autonomy

A final basis for greater attention to futility and rationing is a growing tendency to recognize limits to patient autonomy. Beginning in the early 1960s, the ethical principle of respect for patient autonomy has dominated the field of bioethics, replacing older norms of physician paternalism. The adage that "doctor knows best" was replaced by an ethic of respect for the choices of competent patients. Autonomy was trumpeted by ethicists like Robert Veatch as an overriding ethical value, essentially overriding or canceling out other ethical values, such as beneficence, that may conflict with it.[11]

Although autonomy was a much-needed corrective to medicine, the view that regards autonomy as a "trump card" (i.e., a value that overrides all other values) is increasingly challenged from a variety of sources. And although some continue to insist that patients are entitled to whatever care they want, most bioethicists today recognize that autonomous patients are entitled to choose only from a range of choices that are medically suitable (i.e., supported by professional standards of care). Allan Brett and Laurence McCullough were the first to make a strong case that when a patient seeks to exercise a right to medical care, a necessary condition is that there is either an established or theoretical *medical* basis for the patient's request.[12] In the absence of at least a modicum of medical benefit, they argue, the whole point of the physician-patient interaction disappears.

Others maintain that the moral authority to make decisions regarding futile resuscitation does not rest exclusively with the patient or family, but rather with the community of medicine, which is entitled to establish a professional consensus about the purposes to which their skills will be put. For example, on the basis of a growing literature on the outcomes of medical treatments applied to specific patient groups, physicians and ethicists have argued that physicians should withhold or refrain from offering certain treatments in a range of cases: these include attempted CPR to patients with overwhelming burn injury; patients with no reasonable chance of surviving to discharge from an acute care hospital; terminally ill patients whose lives will be only temporarily prolonged at the cost of unalleviated suffering; severely ill infants whose prognosis is poor and survival questionable; terminally ill patients who have dementia, even those whose families request aggressive treatments.[13]

Another source of challenge to allowing patient autonomy to trump all opposing arguments and values is that health care resources are scarce and may be exhausted long before patients' demands for those resources can be met. Many argue that the health care provider's ethical role now requires balancing justice in the distribution of resources against the responsibility to advocate for individual patients' interests. While some continue to press for health care professionals to devote their energies exclusively to meeting their patients' requests and promoting their patients' welfare, many now hold that physicians do not owe patients a level of resources beyond what patients are entitled to receive, nor must physicians sacrifice their honor, professional integrity, or personal welfare in order to satisfy patients' demands. Others argue that patients' requests should be checked, either by placing physician-patient relationships in the context of institutions that guarantee a fair distribution of resources or by instituting socially sound public policies. Reflecting these sentiments, the President's Commission for the Study of Ethical Problems in Medicine and Biomedical and Behavioral Research, in its 1983 report, *Securing Access to Health Care,* acknowledged that the health care system, like every other system for organizing an activity, "places some limitations on individual choice. . . . Thus, the issue is what kinds of limitations on choice are most consistent with fulfilling society's moral obligation to provide equitable access to health care for all . . . since an adequate level is something less than all care that might be beneficial, patients' choices will be limited to that range unless they are able to pay for care that exceeds adequacy."[14]

The common historical, demographic, economic, and ethical background of futility and rationing makes evident that it will not be possible to keep futility judgment and rationing judgment completely distinct. Whenever the futility of a treatment is debated, its economic cost and context probably lurks in the background of the discussion. This hardly shows, however, that the two concepts *mean* the same thing, or provide the same ethical warrant for withholding or withdrawing treatment. As we shall argue in the next sections, futility and rationing have both common and distinguishing features. Although standards for the rationing of very-low-benefit treatments are likely to be an important part of health care reform, we have argued that futile treatments should not be offered even if they were (hypothetically) cheap and abundant.

Common Features of Futility and Rationing

As illustrated by our patient, Juanita, the tendency for the physician to confuse futility and rationing is not unusual. On the contrary, because attention to futility and rationing has occurred at the same moment in history, the two concepts frequently coexist and may be confused by health care providers and others. Thus, it will be helpful to set forth both the common and distinguishing features.

Futility and rationing share a common ground in situations in which rationing is based on either the quality or likelihood of medical benefit. First, in situations in which rationing assigns a low priority to persons who have the poorest quality of medical outcome, treatment may also be withheld based on a judgment that the *quality* of a particular medical outcome is so extraordinarily poor that it is futile. To state that the quality of outcome is medically futile is to judge that the result achieved by an intervention falls below a minimal medical outcome threshold. That is, if the best result the treatment can achieve is so poor, the treatment should be regarded as futile and not attempted.

Similarly, rationing based on the low likelihood of medical benefit resembles futility assessment based on the poor chance of achieving a certain outcome. Again, medical futility in this sense expresses the idea that the likelihood of achieving an acceptable medical goal is below a threshold considered minimal.

A final resemblance between futility and rationing concerns the manner in which such decisions are reached and implemented. This can range from clearly stated to never articulated, publicly defended to covertly accomplished, and ethically supported to ethically indefensible.

A particularly striking example of the merging of futility and rationing can be seen in the Prioritized List of Health Services (April 1, 2008) of the Oregon Health Plan. At the bottom of the list are diagnostic entities such as "neurologic conditions with no effective treatments or no treatment necessary," and "respiratory conditions with no effective treatments or no treatment necessary," "cardiovascular conditions with no effective treatments or no treatment necessary," "intracranial conditions with no effective treatments or no treatment necessary," and so forth. Because these conditions fall well below the minimum funding level based on budgetary limits, their treatments will not be offered on the grounds of rationing. But clearly, as a matter of definition, any proposed *ineffective* treatments should not be offered anyway on the grounds of medical futility.

Indeed, we are concerned that for some who enter the debate on medical futility, "it's only a matter of money," implying that medicine should take its place next to the "oldest profession" and "do anything" as long as someone is willing to pay for it. The pervasiveness of this perspective was evident in the media coverage of the Baby K case, an anencephalic infant (born with most of her brain, including all higher brain regions, congenitally absent) who was kept alive by medical technology for more than a year (see Chapter 10). The physicians sought to persuade the mother to allow them to stop further medical treatment on the grounds that the baby was deriving no benefit and therefore life prolongation was futile. But the mother went to court demanding that maximal emergency medical care and life prolonging treatment be continued. Media coverage conveyed confusion over the issue. For example, the *New York Times* declared: "Court Order to Treat Baby Prompts a Debate on Ethics." The befuddled subheadline ("At What Point Does Treatment Cease to Be Worth the Expense?") indicated that as far as the newspaper was concerned, the ethical debate was not about whether physicians should be keeping alive a body with no possibility of experiencing any awareness much less any benefit, but rather whether that enterprise was worth the money. This should concern us all. Is this the moral code and professional standard society wishes to assign to medicine? Is this the way physicians see themselves—willing to do anything as long as someone offers to pay for it?

Distinguishing Features of Futility and Rationing

Despite the commonality of meaning between futility and rationing, several distinctions must be noted. Foremost is that futility has no explicit distributive meaning—that is, it does not involve making comparisons across a group of patients, but instead refers to a specific cause-and-effect logic applied to a single patient. Thus, although rationing based on quality or probability of medical benefit partially overlaps with futility, a difference remains. Whereas rationing indicates a priority *among patients who stand to benefit from* scarce resources, futility implies that a particular medical intervention produces an unacceptably low likelihood or quality of benefit *for a particular patient.* Thus, in the case of Juanita, the judgment of medical futility had to come down to this question: Is there at least a reasonable chance that the treatment would achieve an acceptable medical outcome *in this patient,* regardless of who else might deserve it more or derive greater benefit?

A second point of contrast between futility and rationing is that criteria for rationing are far broader in scope than are criteria for defining futility. For example, it might be argued that we should ration based on standards such as age, citizenship, ability to pay, social utility, or equality. However, no one could intelligibly argue that medical treatment is futile on these grounds. The patient could be old or young, a citizen of the United States or Mexico. None of these factors per se affects the potential benefit of the treatment. Strictly speaking, medically futile treatment can be denied only when the patient's particular *medical* circumstances indicate that an expected outcome will fail to meet acceptable goals of medical practice.

A third, and related, point is that ethical rationing must meet standards articulated in theories of distributive justice, namely, theories that purport to tell us what represents a fair distribution of burdens and benefits among different individuals and groups in the society. By contrast, the manner of determining and justifying criteria of medical futility does not make reference to justice theories. Instead, it refers to general professional opinion about such things as medical indications based on reliable empirical data, and community values and goals. In other words, a standard of care regarding medical futility is proposed by the medical profession, then established and confirmed on the basis of a broad consensus among health professionals and others.

A good model to follow here is the evolution to the present definition of death in terms of brain-death criteria. In the 1960s, with the advent of cardiac pacemakers and ventilators, the definition of death became ambiguous and disputed; however, critical ethical debate resulted in a convergence of opinion and consistent policy. We urge that equally vigorous efforts be made to define medical futility. If we fail to exert such efforts and to achieve deliberation and agreement about the definition of medical futility, this will only invite a confusing and, in our opinion, seriously harmful patchwork of case law decisions and inconsistent policies. "Roving strangers" with political motivations will be tempted to run from hospital to hospital and state to state looking for patients like Juanita to use as a means to promoting a singular moral agenda. Such an approach blocks honest public debate and reasoned conversation that can lead to responsible consensus.

A final difference between futility and rationing is that the circumstances of rationing always presuppose scarcity. By contrast, it is possible to argue for denying futile treatment even where a resource is abundant and cheap. For example, even though cough medicine is cheap and abundant, the doctors taking care of Juanita wouldn't even consider prescribing it, for the simple reason that it would not alleviate the patient's medical problems.

The Psychological Roots of Futility and Rationing

One fact is undeniable: We are reluctant to embrace either rationing or futility with open arms. Both are rude awakenings to medicine. Futility forces medicine to come down from its pedestal. Its lesson to medicine is, "Doctor, you are powerless in the face of this calamity." Like Sisyphus, whose repeated efforts were leading nowhere, modern doctors too often continue frantically with medical treatments well past their point of usefulness. Yet such efforts ultimately make no progress in benefiting the patient or curing the disease.

Rationing carries a different message for medicine, but one that also teaches about human limits. It announces loudly, "Doctor, there is something you can do, but we won't let you." Rationing puts someone else in charge. It ties doctors' hands by putting the resources they ask for beyond their reach. Like Odysseus, who heard the sirens but was tied to the mast and prevented from reaching them, the modern doctor is tethered to resource constraints and oversight committees. Yet the analogy between the doctor and Odysseus is not exact, for Odysseus requested to be tied and swore to himself that he would not give in to the sirens' alluring song. Odysseus's restraint therefore showed his self-restraint. Modern physicians, by contrast, are obviously chafing under the restraints imposed on them. Their training teaches them to do everything possible to promote patients' interests. Cost containment is not yet one of the subjects taught in medical school; its lessons come from the outside, causing doctors to feel hemmed in. They often feel inclined, even obligated, to somehow break free. Physicians do not yet define their role as incorporating social responsibilities, or perhaps they do not perceive present resource constraints as just standards for allocating health care.[15]

Just as futility and rationing shake loose the very foundations of medicine by challenging the physician's control and mastery, so too they shake society by challenging its relentless faith in science and medicine. Rationing gives the unmistakable message that not everyone can enjoy the fruits of medicine's labor. (Over the years, during all the many debates on health care reform, many politicians irresponsibly have incanted the word *rationing!* in order to strike fear in the public—as though irrational rationing does not already exist.) Futility reminds society that, despite the great strides science has made, its knowledge and power are ultimately limited. Physicians cannot stave off death forever, doing away with our mortality, but must, in the final analysis, humbly accept death and mortality as part of our shared fate.

These messages are all the more ominous when life-saving medical treatment is at stake. Rationing life-saving treatments implies that even life itself is not of unconditional value; even life is not something we will purchase at any price. Here, rationing's message is not simply that we cannot have it all, but that we must make the ultimate sacrifice. The withdrawal of futile life-sustaining treatments conveys an equally unattractive thought: when life itself is on the line, all of the sophisticated methods of science may be powerless to save it.

As we have already pointed out, the harsh message that futility carries can be softened only when medicine places greater emphasis and value on caring for patients. Saying no to futile treatments is consistent with continuing to nurture and provide comfort to patients. Unfortunately, however, "in American medicine ideals of heroic achievement increasingly have overshadowed the value of nurturance. . . . Technological advances repeatedly have been gained at the expense of the doctor-patient relationship."[16] This state of affairs is not inevitable; recognizing futility challenges physicians to alter it.

With respect to rationing, a similar point is in order. Saying no to costly medical therapies should be compatible with showing respect for persons. Yet this will occur only when rationing is tempered by justice. Rationing can be palatable only provided that it takes place under conditions in which every-one enjoys access to basic services.[17]

The challenge for medicine—indeed, for all of us—is not to recoil by evading hard choices, but instead to realize the limits of medicine in a manner that still preserves, even strengthens, our sense of compassion and community.

CHAPTER SIX

Medical Futility in
a Litigious Society

One summer day in 1988, six-month-old Sammy Linares attended his last birthday party. In the midst of festivities, he choked on a deflated balloon. By the time his father, Rudy Linares, noticed what had happened, the baby was already blue and unconscious. Frantically, the father attempted mouth-to-mouth resuscitation, then picked the child up and ran half a block to a neighborhood fire station for help. There firefighters managed to remove the balloon and continued efforts at resuscitation. But not until the boy was taken by ambulance to the McNeil Hospital emergency room were doctors and nurses able to reestablish the baby's pulse and blood pressure. By then an estimated 20 minutes had elapsed between the baby's asphyxia and the return of his own spontaneous heartbeat.

For the remaining nine months of his life in the pediatric intensive care unit of the Rush Presbyterian St. Luke's Medical Center, the heart continued to beat, but Sammy Linares never regained consciousness. Again and again physicians attempted to withdraw the ventilator, but the baby's brain damage was too severe to allow him to breathe on his own. Reluctantly, the physicians concluded that the baby would never recover consciousness or survive off the ventilator. At this point, Rudy Linares asked that the ventilator be disconnected so that his son could die in peace.

All of the doctors and nurses caring for the baby agreed with the father that there was no point in continuing to keep the permanently unconscious body alive. But even though there were precedents, both in ethics and law, to allow withdrawal of life support under these circumstances,[1] the physicians chose to seek the opinion of the hospital's legal counsel. His response is worth recording: "What we are dealing with here is a legal problem."[2]

Not a medical problem, a legal problem. This astonishing statement reveals how impoverished the notion of medical professional responsibility has become. Before agreeing to discontinue the ventilator, the hospital demanded that the Linares family obtain a court order. Why were the hospital authorities unwilling to go to court themselves if they truly believed in the appropriateness of the request and were simply seeking legal protection? The most likely explanation is that the best interests of the patient were overshadowed by the hospital's concern for its own public image. The Linares family had already cost the state's Medicaid program over a half million dollars. Wouldn't the hospital be vulnerable to the tabloid press if it were sensationalized as a killer of welfare babies? Rather than risk its reputation, the hospital was prepared to keep the unconscious baby alive indefinitely.

Meanwhile, Rudy Linares kept repeating his request that the baby be allowed to die in peace. Once, while visiting his son in the middle of the night, he disconnected the ventilator himself, but security guards wrestled him to the ground and the medical staff reconnected the machine.

After nine months the distraught father took a more desperate step in carrying out his wishes. Following one of their visits, he sent his wife away and suddenly produced a gun. Holding the intensive care unit staff at bay and saying, "I'm not here to hurt anyone," he disconnected his son's respirator and waited for the boy to die. As proof that he meant no harm, he allowed the hospital staff to remove three other patients from the intensive care unit. Then, after confirming the baby's death with a stethoscope that a physician slid across the floor, Rudy Linares surrendered to police.

To the hospital administration's astonishment, when the story reached the press they had so feared, the public outrage was directed against them—not against Mr. Linares. The state's attorney filed a murder complaint, requiring Rudy Linares to undergo a psychiatric evaluation as a condition of his bond, but a grand jury refused to issue a homicide indictment. In the end Rudy Linares was found guilty only of a misdemeanor weapons charge. Indeed, many of us in the field of bioethics thought that the only crime for which Mr. Linares could be found guilty was practicing medicine without a license. For Mr. Linares, in his own clumsy, desperate way, was trying to do what all the doctors and nurses wanted to do—*thought they ought to do*—but failed to do.

Fear of Lawyers

In this chapter we explore the interactions of medicine and the law, particularly with respect to establishing standards of care determining medical futility. But first we must acknowledge the immense presence of the law in contemporary American society. A few statistics can serve. Between 1960 and 1990 the number of lawyers in this country nearly tripled, from 260,000 to 756,000. According to the American Bar Association there are currently about 1.1 million lawyers practicing in the United States. Although the ratio of lawyers to the general population remained fairly constant at about 120 per 100,000 Americans until 1970, now that ratio is about 300 lawyers per 100,000—the highest in the world.[3] In the area of health care, lawyers have not only contributed to the practice commonly known as "defensive medicine," but have influenced every aspect of health care delivery. As *Washington Post* reporter Jeffrey H. Birnbaum wrote in 2005: "To the great growth industries of America such as health care and home building add one more: influence peddling. The number of registered lobbyists in Washington has more than doubled since 2000 to more than 34,750 while the amount the lobbyists charge their new clients has increased as much as 100 percent."[4] During the battle over health care reform in 2009, drug companies alone spent more than $245 million, more than any other single industry has ever spent on any other single issue. Ironically, new regulations under the Obama administration have driven many lobbyists (most of them lawyers, who are skilled at circumventing restrictions) underground. "All the increasing restrictions on lobbyists are a disincentive to be a lobbyist, and those who think they can deregister are eagerly doing so," said Jan Baran, a "veteran political lawyer."[5]

Whether or not the medical malpractice system adversely influences the behavior of physicians, prompting them to prescribe tests and treatments whose principal aim is to protect themselves from lawsuits rather than protect their patients from disease, is a subject of continuing controversy. Unfortunately, the latest empirical evidence suggests that fear of liability does distort the practice of medicine. In one recent study, more than 90 percent of physicians report ordering tests, performing diagnostic procedures, and referring patients for consultation not as a matter of medical judgment but out of fear of being sued.[6] And although costs incurred and harm caused by overuse cannot be separated easily from other influences (such as financial incentives and restrictions, patients' preferences for aggressive treatments, requirements of peer review organizations, and prevailing notions of safety and efficacy), analysts long ago agreed that "defensive medicine is a real phenomenon accounting for at least some marginal or unnecessary care."[7]

Rather than improving medical care, the current malpractice system actually perpetuates repetition of medical errors because the adversarial nature of litigation induces a so-called culture of silence in physicians eager to shield themselves from liability.[8] And although jury awards, settlements, and administrative costs by themselves amount to less than $10 billion a year—less than one-half of a percentage point of medical spending—the consequences of this kind of wasteful treatment extend beyond these damages and are estimated to amount to as much as $60 billion a year, or about 3 percent of overall medical spending.[9]

For example, in 1988, the American College of Obstetricians and Gynecologists dropped its long-standing policy requiring electronic fetal monitoring (EFM) of all pregnant women and declared that it was no longer medically necessary for the majority of low-risk women. Subsequent studies and consensus statements supported this recommendation and even noted that EFM was associated with an increased rate of potentially hazardous operative interventions, including forceps use and cesarean delivery, without improving infant outcomes.[10] Even so, the majority of obstetricians continue to use this expensive technology "despite overwhelming evidence that it does not improve neonatal mortality and morbidity rates."[11] Why? According to Peter Huber, an expert on liability law, "Lawyers have discovered in EFM the perfect technological wand to wave before juries."[12] Not long ago the courts showed an infatuation with outright fraudulent treatments, particularly those purported to be cancer cures, like Laetrile, immunoaugmentive therapy, and thermography. A review of court cases initiated by patients seeking insurance coverage for the costs of these treatments revealed that, rather than relying on peer-reviewed scientific literature, interpreted if necessary by impartial experts, the courts often relied on "testimony by practitioners who either were the attending physician of the insured or had a vested interest in coverage of the subject procedures."[13] Astonishingly, testimonies tainted by conflict of interest that would disqualify any claim of scientific objectivity *took precedence* in these legal deliberations.

Is it any wonder that physicians seeking to practice careful, rational medicine despaired of achieving their goal in a legal environment so appallingly misguided at times in scientific and medical matters? Fortunately, all this may be changing as a result of the U.S. Supreme Court decision *Daubert v. Merrell Dow*, which assigns to the trial judge "the task of ensuring that an expert's testimony both rests on a reliable foundation and is relevant to the task at hand."[14] The *Daubert* decision now seems to have become the standard for toxic tort cases across the nation, allowing courts to determine with far more precision than before when expert evidence is valid and when it is not. In several important trials, *Daubert* was a crucial case for ensuring that judges did not allow junk science, and particularly junk medicine, in their courtrooms.[15]

A survey of hospitals in New York State revealed the curious finding that the number of caesarean sections performed in the different hospitals varied directly with the number of malpractice claims. Because there was no significant association between caesarean deliveries and malpractice claims for individual physicians *within* each hospital, the researchers concluded that the quality of practice was not leading to the malpractice claims, but rather the other way around: the physicians' *fear* of malpractice suits was leading them to increase their tendency to perform the surgical procedure.[16]

Huber points out that "in technology-intensive professions like medicine or aviation, there will *always* be a spare high-tech instrument, heroic procedure, or exotic medicine lying around that could have been tried, that might conceivably have made things turn out better." He adds caustically: "The cautionary CAT scan or caesarean, the amniocentesis, blood test, or fetal monitor can be certified as essential by lawyers much faster than by scientists. These tests and gadgets then accumulate in the cockpit and the operating theater, because not having them on hand has become legally risky. As the unnecessary or unreliable tests and technologies multiply, so do the opportunities for ignoring them in the heat of a crisis. Which creates opportunities for still more legal action."[17]

It is vital that society recognize this dilemma: the medical profession's effort to practice a reasonable, commonsense, (not to mention cost-effective), medicine by eliminating unnecessary tests and futile treatments (based on empirical evidence) leaves the profession vulnerable to legal attack, even if only in rare and exceptional cases. This conflict can harm patients and families most directly, but it also imposes costs on society and medicine. Physicians themselves become complicit in producing tragic and unfortunate medical outcomes. It also illustrates the importance of educating the public (and juries) that the reasonable practice of medicine does not include using every conceivable test or treatment in every situation. To do so is to make an unwise tradeoff: exchanging the small chance that a benefit might be missed for the greater chance that much harm will result, through adverse effects and injuries caused by medical tests and treatments spurred by false positive findings, as well as because of the generally diminished quality of life that is so often a by-product of intensive medical treatment. This caution applies as well to the area of screening, where a recent review of breast and prostate cancer outcomes suggests that "screening may be increasing the burden of low-risk cancers without significantly reducing the burden of more aggressively growing cancers and therefore not resulting in the anticipated reduction in cancer mortality."[18] Sadly, this sensible caution based on empirical evidence was greeted with outrage by many Americans who equate more (and more expensive) with better.[19] Will this opposition to good medical practice continue and hinder efforts at health care reform?

This is not an idle speculation. When attempts were made to study the effectiveness of high-dose chemotherapy with bone marrow transplantation to treat breast cancer they ran up against unexpected obstacles. For many years there was no good empirical evidence based on randomized control trials that the controversial, burdensome, and highly expensive treatment was more effective than conventional chemotherapy. Even so, many patients hired lawyers to force insurance companies to pay for the treatment.[20] Patients who had metastatic breast cancer were unwilling to participate in clinical trials or wait for their results. They wanted the new, unproven treatment *now* and wanted it fully covered by insurance. One writer described the project as illustrating the complexity of doing research "in an arena of divided physicians, desperate patients, reluctant insurers, aggressive lawyers and revenue-hungry hospitals." But in large part, said the writer, the blame falls on physicians who "lack the courage to say no to patients."[21] Alas, the consequence of this lack of courage was immense suffering during the 1980s and 1990s by an estimated 30,000 thousand women who underwent what turned out to be a futile treatment when at last definitive randomized control trials showed that it provided no improvement in lifespan over conventional chemotherapy.[22]

As members of hospital ethics committees, both of us have been involved in formulating policies for withholding and withdrawing treatment. This can provoke considerable anxiety among physicians. For example, when one hospital ethics committee completed a carefully drafted policy and submitted it to the various clinical services for their review, one physician demanded that the ethics consultant run the policy draft past some "aggressive lawyers" to see where the loopholes were. To his credit the first lawyer responded, without even looking at the policy, that "physicians shouldn't be practicing medicine to avoid lawsuits, they should do what is best for the patient." The ethics consultant returned with this advice to the committee, and the policy was adopted without further ado.

Fears of the Law and Legal Myths

It is ironic that doctors have sometimes forced patients and families to accept unwanted or inappropriate life-prolonging treatments out of misplaced fear of legal liability. As professor of philosophy and clinical ethics Lance Stell points out, "From *Quinlan* [in 1976] to the present, our courts have rejected the notion that physicians have a duty to preserve biological existence per se."[23] In the *Quinlan* decision, the court asserted that "the focal point of decision should be the prognosis as to the reasonable possibility of return to cognitive and sapient life, as distinguished from the forced continuance of the biological vegetative existence."[24] It is worth drawing attention to the word *reasonable*, which performs invaluable service in U.S. jurisprudence and might serve as a guide to medical practice. In the law, even when the defendant's life hangs in the balance, say, at a trial for murder, the jury is admonished to base its conviction on evidence persuasive not beyond all doubt but beyond all *reasonable* doubt. Reasonableness tempers judgment. Similarly, physicians should also temper their judgments; they are obligated to apply their skills not if there is any miraculous chance of success but where there is a *reasonable* chance of success.

It is worth repeating that there has never been a single criminal conviction of a physician for withdrawing life-sustaining treatment, and only one conviction of a physician who deliberately acted to end the life of a patient—the notorious "Dr. Death" (Dr. Kevorkian), whom numerous juries refused to convict even when he openly testified that he had set up an apparatus designed to allow a patient to kill himself. For all the scare stories that circulate in doctors' lounges, the reasoned medical decision to allow a patient to die is not considered medical negligence by the courts and threatened with astronomical awards. In a paper sharply critical of the medical and legal professions, whose "serious misunderstanding of the law can lead to tragic results for physicians, health care institutions, patients, and families," professor of law and ethicist Alan Meisel summarizes eight "myths about what the law permits concerning the termination of life support."[25]

Myth 1: "Anything that is not specifically permitted by law is prohibited." This myth, Meisel says, "is held dear not only by some health care professionals, but by the general public and by many people who ought to know better—namely lawyers." This led to the tragedy of the Linares case, as indeed the hospital counsel testified: "I told the medical staff there was a possibility they would face criminal charges." Proffering this advice, the attorney played the role of one of the "paid paranoids whose perceived function it is to conjure up worst-case hypothetical scenarios and accordingly to render the most conservative, risk-averse advice to their clients."[26]

But, as lawyer Lawrence J. Nelson and physician Ronald E. Cranford point out, "An experienced and knowledgeable attorney, particularly one dealing with physicians and hospitals, should construct his or her advice on probabilities, not abstract possibilities. The practical probability in this case of a physician being prosecuted for murder was remote to the point of being nonexistent, fundamentally because the law and the facts of this situation would not support even a vaguely plausible prosecution for unlawful, malicious killing."[27]

If ignorance of the law is found among lawyers, it seems to be widespread among physicians. Indeed, ignorance of the law, along with misguided notions that equate withholding every last means of prolonging terminal life with killing, was prevalent among more than 700 physicians surveyed by the Institute for Medical Humanities in Galveston.[28] Ultimately, of course, health professionals, not lawyers, treat patients. So, not unreasonably, the researchers expressed concern over the inevitable consequences of these attitudes among physicians—unnecessary suffering of patients and families and inappropriate use of futile or scarce resources.

Myth 2: "Termination of life support is murder or suicide." As we have noted already, court decisions around the country, including the U.S. Supreme Court's *Cruzan* decision, make clear that termination of inappropriate or unwanted life support in a medical setting is neither murder nor suicide if the physician has acted after appropriate consultation with colleagues, discussions with the patient or surrogate, and in the event of disagreement, with an ethics committee. The position the courts take is that removal of life-sustaining treatment under these circumstances merely allows nature to take its course and that the patient's illness, not the treatment removal, causes death.

Myth 3: "A patient must be terminally ill for life support to be stopped." Although the validity of advance directives (living wills and durable powers of attorney for health care) was in the past limited in many states to the final period of terminal illness, today advance directives apply to a wider range of situations and treatments. In particular, the U.S. Supreme Court's *Cruzan* decision, although permitting a state to apply any evidentiary standard it sees fit, granted competent patients or their legal surrogates the right to refuse *any* treatment, including nutrition and hydration, regardless of whether they have a terminal illness. And in fact many courts have permitted withdrawal of treatment in a variety of instances short of terminal illness, including severe cerebral palsy, temporary uterine bleeding, kidney failure requiring renal dialysis, persistent vegetative state, and quadriplegia. Moreover, patients who are aware and have the capacity to make decisions for themselves have a legal and ethical right to refuse any treatments, even life-sustaining treatments, either orally or in writing at any time.

Myth 4: "It is permissible to terminate extraordinary treatments, but not ordinary ones." The distinction between ordinary and extraordinary treatments has evaporated as medical technology becomes more and more ordinary. Once, maintaining patients through feeding tubes was considered extraordinary; now there are those who argue that such feeding tubes represent basic life support. Today, attempted CPR, mechanical ventilation, renal dialysis, and the entire panoply of intensive-care unit treatments are undertaken as a matter of course in seriously ill patients. Are such treatments ordinary or extraordinary? In the tradition of Catholic moral theology, extraordinary treatments were regarded as those that provided no benefit and whose burdens were excessive. Such a distinction can apply to even the simplest measures. Even intravenous fluids can be regarded as extraordinary if they do nothing but maintain an unconscious or incurably suffering patient.

Today, ethicists and courts tend to measure treatments not in terms of ordinary versus extraordinary, but in terms of *proportionality of benefits versus burdens*. That is, does the treatment, whatever it is, result overall in a balance of benefits (chance of saving cognitive, sapient life or restoring function or alleviating suffering) over burdens (pain, suffering, loss of dignity, and costs)?

Are the burdens imposed proportionate to the benefits gained? For example, is not the prolongation of life by only a few days *dis*proportionate to the imposition of great suffering and expenditure of tens of thousands of dollars—as occurs today in many intensive care units around the country? In the case of medical futility, the intervention under consideration does not produce any significant benefit; thus, the need to weigh benefits against burdens does not arise. Yet in many other situations benefits and burdens must be considered in tandem in precisely this manner.

Myth 5: "It is permissible to withhold treatment but, once started, it must be continued." Although health care providers and families recognize that emotionally it is sometimes more difficult to discontinue a treatment that has been started, the law has clearly followed the lead of *Barber v. Los Angeles County Superior Court,* which noted that any treatment may be viewed in terms of whether or not the next application of that treatment is likely to benefit the patient.[29] The *Barber* decision deliberately drew no distinction between withholding a ventilator or discontinuing a ventilator in a patient for whom this machine provides no benefit. Obviously, there is a practical as well as theoretical value to equating withholding and withdrawing futile treatments. Physicians who are fearful of having to "pull the plug" at some later time might be tempted to avoid starting a desperate life-saving procedure. Unfortunately, this misguided fear might lead them to make hasty decisions with insufficient knowledge or time to reflect and, paradoxically, to *withhold* potentially beneficial treatments. For example, a patient brought into the emergency room might be an uncertain candidate for cardiopulmonary resuscitation or immediate ventilation. If the physician were to start these procedures and if they turned out to be beneficial, they could of course be continued. If, on the other hand, they turned out to be useless or harmful, they could *then* be discontinued. But what if the physician—to avoid facing difficult decisions—never gave the patient a "fighting chance"?

Myth 6: "Stopping tube feeding is legally different from stopping other treatments." The usual concern of those who seek to distinguish tube feeding from other forms of medical treatment is that patients should not be allowed to "starve to death." Yet as clinical experience has evolved (and as we have discussed in previous chapters), health professionals have learned that forcing artificial nutrition and hydration into patients who are terminally ill often adds to their suffering rather than reducing it.[30] Moreover, artificially imposing any life-prolonging interventions beyond the patient's own choice runs the risk of violating that patient's autonomy. Thus, throughout this country and finally in the U.S. Supreme Court *Cruzan* decision, most courts have held that there is no legal distinction between the termination of artificial nutrition and hydration and other forms of treatment. At this point we must note that the Terri Schiavo case has spurred a disturbing new tactic: a coalition of "right-to-life" activists—conservative Catholics and politicians, evangelicals, and splinter groups from disability rights organizations—are directing their efforts in the courts and state legislatures seeking laws that prohibit withdrawal of tube feedings under any circumstance, permit pharmacists to refrain from providing birth control medications, and invalidate advance directives, such as living wills.[31] Such efforts threaten to undermine the legitimate exercise of patient autonomy: the right to choose from among medically effective and beneficial options. They also threaten the legitimate exercise of professional ethics: the physician's obligation to offer (or continue) only those treatments that are shown to benefit the patient.

Myth 7: "Termination of life support requires going to court." The persistence of this common misperception attests to the pervasive power of the "litigious society." It is a notion all the more absurd—if the word were not too inexpressive of the suffering caused—when one contemplates the multitude of decisions made every day by physicians that in effect terminate life-sustaining treatments. Every time a surgeon decides against performing a desperate operation, the surgeon has made a choice based on the odds that the patient will die versus the possibility that the operation will succeed. Every time a physician prescribes high doses of a narcotic to alleviate pain in a dying patient, the physician has chosen a course of action that might shorten a patient's life. In other words, the daily practice of medicine has always involved choosing *alternatives* to prolonging patients' lives. The courts are not called on to participate in these treatment choices. But with the advent of high technology has come the fearsome phrase "pulling the plug," as though tubes and wires and electrical power possess ethical dimensions by themselves. The myth that one must go to court before terminating life support (purveyed even by lawyers themselves, as was so tragically evident in the Linares case) is belied by the daily experience of health providers in hospitals, nursing homes, and hospices. Efforts at prolonging the life of dying patients are routinely and humanely reduced in favor of palliation, and judicial involvement in these decisions is routinely absent.

Notwithstanding the countless times physicians have terminated life support (and it is impossible to know how many times actions have been brought against physicians in unrecorded lower court cases), only once in this highly litigious country has a physician been found criminally guilty for terminating life support—and then only after defiantly showing himself performing it on the television program *60 Minutes*. One landmark decision acknowledged: "Courts are not the proper place to resolve the agonizing personal problems that underlie these cases. Our legal system cannot replace the more intimate struggle that must be borne by the patient, those caring for the patient, and those who care about the patient."[32] And as Meisel, himself, laments, "Litigation adds trial to tribulation, both literally and figuratively. There are all sorts of costs, and in advance they are incalculable. Litigation is expensive and emotionally draining (sometimes unimaginably so), primarily because it is also time-consuming—so time-consuming that in many end of life cases the patient expires before the litigation does. And in the end, litigation is a blunt instrument for the resolution of disputes."[33]

Finally, we note that even when patients or loved ones initially insist on treatment, open and honest communication generally limits the risk that a lawsuit will be brought and therefore reduces the need for judicial involvement as a procedural safeguard. When patients and family members already agree, or are eventually persuaded, to allow futile treatments to be withheld or withdrawn, the legal exposure of health professionals is even more limited and the appropriateness of obtaining a court ruling is even more doubtful.

Myth 8: "Living wills are not legal." By this Meisel refers to the fears of many physicians that if the patient is no longer capable of participating in the process of making treatment decisions personally, all other means of conveying the patient's wishes are legally suspect. Although considerable efforts are routinely made to encourage patients to execute "advance directives"—documents that specify in writing a patient's wishes (living wills) or designate a person to act as a proxy decision-maker (durable power of attorney for health care)—these documents are proving to be blunt tools, offering inadequate remedies in many complex medical situations.[34]

The challenges are numerous. First, because people find it difficult to contemplate or discuss the end of their lives, only a small percentage of patients—even among those with life-threatening illness such as metastatic cancer—ever execute advance directives.[35] Second, patients turn out to be inconsistent and somewhat unstable in their treatment preferences. Not surprisingly, they change their minds. One obvious explanation for this is that patients (who usually lack a medical education) are rarely fully knowledgeable about treatments and their consequences in advance. If you ask a patient, "Do you want us to get your heart going again if it stops?" almost universally the patient will answer, "Of course." It sounds so easy, why not? (One colleague sarcastically suggested that the question might better be phrased: "If you die, do you want us to bring you back to life?") But a patient may arrive at a completely different decision when informed that attempted cardiopulmonary resuscitation could involve shocking the heart with high-voltage electricity; involves forceful, even violent, efforts at compressing the chest cage to the point of fracturing ribs; usually requires thrusting a tube into the trachea and placement on a mechanical ventilator; and often results in outcomes that, in the presence of serious disease like cancer, are rarely successful and may end with the patient's having serious brain damage. Moreover, even the most fully informed patients facing critical illness may change their minds, and no one, neither patient nor physician, can predict with certainty how a person will feel in the future.

A further, potentially more serious, problem with advance directives is that a physician may demand a legal document before acting on a patient's wishes, or before withdrawing obviously futile treatment. Our concern is that in a litigious society, even a patient's authentic expressions of preferences to a physician, family member, or close friend will not be considered sufficient to represent the patient's wishes. Such oral or even written statements may be ignored if they are not expressed in "legal" documents. As noted below, in at least three states—Missouri, New York, and California—the requirement that there be "clear and convincing" evidence of a patient's treatment wishes has led to judicial travesties.

Judges and Medicine

In Chapter 1, we described the agonizing struggle the Cruzan family had to go through to withdraw life support from their permanently unconscious daughter because the state of Missouri would not recognize the authority of her family to speak on her behalf. And in Chapter 8 we describe the case of Mary O'Connor in New York, a nearly unconscious elderly woman with dementia, whose relative was prevented from achieving the withdrawal of the patient's feeding tube because the patient had not specifically predicted her own circumstances. This occurred despite repeated requests by the patient, who had been a hospital worker, that she not be kept alive in circumstances similar to those of the many patients she had seen. All her previous statements were discounted by New York's highest court as not fulfilling the "clear and convincing" standard of evidence.

In the case of Robert Wendland, who had been unconscious for over a year before remaining another five years in a minimally conscious state, the California Supreme Court refused to allow his wife of 20 years to interpret the prior statements he made to family members nor his repeatedly ripping out a surgically implanted feeding tube as his desire not to be kept alive by this artificial means.[36] Unfortunately for Mr. Wendland, his prior statements did not meet the standards set by the California justices in that they did not "clearly illustrate a serious, well thought out, consistent decision to refuse treatment under these exact circumstances, or circumstances highly similar to the current situation." As one of us commented, "Unfortunately the justices seemed to know little about the reality of human behavior in these matters. . . . Not many laypersons have the knowledge or foresight to express their end-of-life wishes in exact detail and anticipate 'exact circumstances.' One entire group, the developmentally disabled from birth or childhood, could never meet the standard. As for Robert Wendland, by the time he was under medical care he was incapable of nominating a surrogate decision maker or orally informing his supervising physician about his 'specific health-care instructions.'"[37] Nearly eight years after his injury, the bedfast, incommunicative Mr. Wendland died, his feeding tube securely in place.

In all three cases, the lives of these patients were prolonged as much by the law as by medicine. They illustrate therefore that the practice of "defensive medicine" is not always based on misplaced fears, but is also imposed by unrealistic legal standards. Sadly, though, it is not the physician who suffers the burdens of these unrealistic legal standards so much as the patient.

The problems associated with defensive medicine are not new. When one of the authors was a medical intern in the late 1950s he saw patient after patient admitted to the private service with vague—and usually psychosomatic—abdominal pains who were given what the house staff disparagingly called "the complete radio-opaque work-up": upper GI series, barium enema, intravenous pyelogram, and gall bladder X-ray. A mere few minutes spent with these patients were enough to predict that all the studies would be negative—and the private physician knew they would be. Still, the effort to reassure the patient without performing the ceremony of tests ("Doctor, can you be absolutely *sure* there's no cancer in there?") and the fear that lurking behind every complaint was a potential lawsuit were enough to overturn all the lectures of medical school. ("Listen to the patient. He is telling you the diagnosis.")

Today the physician (and the hapless patient) caught up in the quest for foolproof medicine confront a technology that is even more formidable, involving penetrations and infusions into every recess of the body, and treatments that are often far more monstrous even as they are more powerful, rendering the patient hairless, marrowless, and immunologically helpless. And every day the problem becomes more disquieting. As patients continue to expect more from medicine, they look more to the law. They expect medicine to fulfill their hopes, and when medicine fails, they somehow expect redress through the courts, as though lawyers and juries can provide what is desired: the miraculous restoration of health and preservation of life. Indeed, only at the very end of life has the law so far acknowledged that perhaps death *is* inevitable. But how long will medicine enjoy even this respite? Understandably, we hail—and even more, anticipate—the seemingly endless supply of miracles from modern medicine. But as scientific optimism lurches forward, will the law be far behind?[38]

CHAPTER SEVEN

Ethical Implications
of Medical Futility

In Chapter 6 we noted that physicians and hospitals have sometimes forced patients to undergo futile treatments out of a misplaced fear of legal liability. If we look back to the decades of the 1970s and 1980s, we find that the ethical cases gaining attention most typically dealt with situations of this sort: patients or families wished to withdraw treatment, but the health care institution either felt it was improper to do so or wanted legal immunity first. So, for example, in *Quinlan*, the family requested that treatment be stopped despite misgivings on the part of the institution (the court decided in favor of the family). Likewise, in a host of similar cases (*Saikewicz*, 1977; *Brophy*, 1985; *Cruzan*, 1990), families requested that treatment be stopped but were thwarted by health care institutions and physicians who were concerned about the legality of meeting such a request.[1]

During the 1990s, we witnessed a reversal of this trend. Increasingly, cases dealt with situations in which the patient, or more often the family, wished to do everything possible for a loved one, while the medical team or hospital sought to end futile treatments. Thus, in the Wanglie case (introduced in Chapter 4), the family wished to continue life-sustaining treatment of an

86-year-old woman in a persistent vegetative state over the objections of doctors at Hennepin County Medical Center, who wanted the patient removed from the ventilator. Mr. Wanglie believed that life should be maintained as long as possible, no matter what the circumstances and asserted that his wife, Helga Wanglie, shared this belief. Similarly, in other cases that took place during this time, such as the anencephalic Baby K (1994) and the permanently unconscious 71-year-old Catherine Gilgunn (1995) it was the medical team or the hospital that wanted to stop treatment, while the family insisted on pressing on with futile treatments. The Gilgunn case became the first case in which a jury agreed that "it was appropriate for the treating physician—even over the family's vehement protests—to withhold interventions deemed by the physician to be 'futile.' "[2]

This trend continued more recently, in 2005, in the case of Terri Schiavo (see Chapter 1), but with a slightly different twist. In *Schiavo*, we witnessed a family that was deeply divided. While the patient's husband sought to end artificial nutrition and hydration, her parents wished to continue it. The trend we are describing suggests to us that hospitals and medical teams are moving away from an earlier tendency to press for futile treatments. Families, while sometimes divided as in *Schiavo*, are beginning to come to grips with the very difficult reality that stopping life-sustaining measures can be the most humane course.

In this chapter we explore the ethical responsibilities of physicians when a treatment is determined to be futile. Before we begin, however, we need to consider and dispense with an important objection. One objection to any claim that physicians should not offer futile treatment is to raise the specter of medical uncertainty. Realistically, we have to ask, If futility refers to a treatment that doesn't work, how do we *know* it doesn't work? That is, how often should physicians try to achieve a desired medical outcome before they draw conclusions about the success or failure of their efforts? As we pointed out, physicians could try a million times to resuscitate a cadaver and still be vulnerable to the claim that maybe the next time they will succeed. But nowhere in medicine is the physician absolutely certain that a treatment will succeed or fail. Rather, medical practice emerges out of empirical experience, sometimes based on accurate and reliable clinical research, and many times, unfortunately, based on hearsay, habit, and false and unreliable claims.

Partly because physicians can "never say never," partly because of the seduction of modern technology, and partly out of the misplaced fear of litigation, physicians have shown an increasing tendency to undertake treatments that have no realistic expectation of success. As we said earlier, we have to remember the denominator. If physicians submit to demands that cardiopulmonary resuscitation be attempted even if there's only a one in a hundred chance of success, they are literally and cruelly agreeing to attempt a procedure in which 99 patients will be subjected to a brutal death in pursuit of the minute chance that one patient will survive. For this reason, we have articulated commonsense criteria for defining medical futility.

We propose that a treatment should be regarded as medically futile if empirical data have shown that it has not worked in the last 100 cases, or if the treatment fails to restore consciousness or alleviate total dependence for survival on medical treatments available only in the acute care hospital setting. This definition recognizes that the goal of medicine is not merely to maintain a patient in a condition that constitutes total entrapment in the illness and treatment but rather one that enables the patient to achieve a level of health that permits the pursuit of life goals, however limited, outside the walls of the hospital. At the very least, the outcome to be achieved—which is the endpoint of every published important life-sustaining treatment trial—is discharge from the hospital.

This definition provides clear end points and encourages the profession to review data from the past and perform prospective clinical research to determine not only which treatments work but also which treatments do not.[3] Both kinds of information are essential for doctors and patients to decide when to say yes and when to say no to medical treatments.

In this chapter we consider questions such as the following: How should we understand the ethical obligations of physicians when a treatment is shown, on the basis of empirical evidence, to be medically futile? What should a responsible physician do and not do? Are physicians ethically allowed to decide on their own whether or not to offer a futile treatment? Should the medical profession as a whole set forth standards to guide or require compliance? Finally, what is the role of patients and society? What are the possible consequences and risks of granting the authority to make futility judgments to any of the above parties? All these questions require an examination of the ethical implications of medical futility—an examination not of definitions or data, but of values and actions. Exploring the ethical arguments surrounding medical futility inevitably involves reexamining the very nature of the doctor-patient relationship, particularly the limits of this relationship and the limits of what we can expect from medicine and the physician.

We begin with the case of Arthur Tanney (not his real name), a 69-year-old man admitted for treatment of metastatic carcinoma of the colon. Upon admission to the hospital, he was informed of his rights under the Patient Self-Determination Act to refuse any unwanted treatments. Before beginning chemotherapy, Mr. Tanney was informed by Dr. Garland (not her real name) of the anticipated toxicity of the treatment and of the limited chance of good-quality and sustained response to treatment. Furthermore, Dr. Garland told Mr. Tanney that in the event of a cardiac arrest during his treatment program, she would not attempt cardiopulmonary resuscitation. She explained that in patients with metastatic cancer, attempting CPR had a negligible chance of success and an almost certain chance of prolonging suffering before a patient died in the intensive care unit. In other words, CPR would be futile. Mr. Tanney accepted Dr. Garland's decision and a Do Not Attempt Resuscitation (DNAR) order was written.

The night after chemotherapy was started, Mr. Tanney developed periods of irregular heartbeat. The physician on duty that night, Dr. Sylvester (also not his real name), rushed to the bedside and, while initiating treatment and arranging immediate transfer to the coronary care unit (CCU), told Mr. Tanney he would attempt CPR if his heart stopped beating effectively. Mr. Tanney nodded in apparent agreement. Shortly thereafter Mr. Tanney underwent a cardiac arrest, and Dr. Sylvester immediately started efforts at CPR. These efforts failed, and the patient died. The next day at case conference, Dr. Sylvester and Dr. Garland, as well as several other physicians, engaged in heated debate over whether CPR should have been attempted. Dr. Sylvester asserted that it was his personal belief that physicians had a duty to preserve life whenever possible. Dr. Garland countered that a doctor's personal belief should not override a patient's preference. She argued that the patient had previously agreed to a DNAR order. Dr. Sylvester countered that by nodding agreement, the patient had changed his mind.

A conference was arranged, and one of us was asked to join the group. During this conference it became apparent that all the physicians were acquainted with a medical journal article that had recently summarized CPR outcomes in several medical centers. The article reported that when CPR was required and attempted in a total of 117 patients with metastatic cancer, not one patient survived to hospital discharge.[4] The author of the report concluded that such treatment was futile and should not be attempted.

The case conference debate then evolved from the question of whether CPR have been attempted in Mr. Tanney to what physicians should do when considering *any* treatment that is likely to fail. Several views were aired, including the following: (1) Dr. Sylvester was ethically *permitted* to refrain from attempting CPR, but he was also ethically permitted to perform it. In other words, in the presence of a clinical situation in which treatment is futile, it is completely up to the individual physician to act as he or she wishes. (2) Dr. Sylvester should have been *encouraged* not to attempt CPR on Mr. Tanney. That is, the findings of the study and the recommendation by the author not to attempt CPR might be considered an ethical guideline that physicians are urged, but not required, to follow. (3) Finally, once CPR was shown to be futile, Dr. Sylvester was ethically *required* as a matter of professional duty to refrain from attempting it.

In weighing these distinct views, several comparisons might prove helpful. In the first instance, allowing Dr. Sylvester to make an individual decision about attempting CPR on a patient with metastatic cancer would be ethically analogous to allowing an obstetrics and gynecology physician to decide whether or not to meet a woman's request to perform therapeutic abortion. The medical profession, while accepting abortion as a legal choice for all women, takes an ethically neutral stance and allows individual physicians to refuse to perform the procedure as a matter of personal conscience. Any physician not complying with a patient's request for abortion therefore would not be acting unethically.

In the second instance, encouraging but not requiring Dr. Sylvester to refrain from attempting CPR is analogous to a physician's decision to support life in patients with permanent vegetative state. Several professional societies have recommended against maintaining patients in permanent vegetative state, yet physicians are not ethically or legally bound to follow these advisory recommendations.[5] Similarly, Dr. Sylvester would be ethically free to attempt CPR in Mr. Tanney; however, refraining from CPR would be regarded as an ethically preferable course.

In the third instance the ethical equivalent is the treatment of patients with human immunodeficiency virus (HIV) infection. The medical profession has specifically mandated that it is the duty of all physicians not to discriminate against patients on the basis of their HIV status. Therefore, a physician who refuses to treat a patient simply because the patient has this condition would violate an ethical duty. Similarly, then, attempting CPR in patients with metastatic cancer would be considered *prima facie* wrong for all physicians by virtue of violating professional standards against applying futile treatments to patients. By this standard, Dr. Sylvester's effort was wrong even though Mr. Tanney had requested CPR, because physicians are generally not entitled to breach standards of their profession.

Addressing these three viewpoints provides the central focus for this chapter. In what follows we proceed stepwise. First, we argue that physicians are ordinarily ethically *permitted* to refrain from offering or continuing futile treatment. Then we make the stronger point that physicians should generally be *encouraged* to omit futile therapies. Finally, we present the still stronger case that physicians are generally ethically *required* to decline the use of futile interventions.

The Ends of Medicine

Some have argued that medicine has no "core" values.[6] If this is true, then talking about integrity in medicine is meaningless because medicine has no essential values that physicians must uphold. Alternatively, it may be argued that medicine stands not for a single morality, but rather multiple moralities, constituting "many medicines."[7] If that is the case, then the idea of integrity in medicine is ambiguous. To say that a physician ought to uphold medicine's values leaves the physician to wonder which medical morality to uphold.

Yet these approaches belie the entire history of medicine, as we understand it.[8] From Hippocrates to the present, the practice of medicine has been based on the value and duty of *beneficence*, or doing good for the patient. In Chapter 1 we described the historic traditions of medicine that underlie our proposal that medical interventions be regarded as futile when the odds of achieving a medical goal are exceedingly slim or when the quality of the outcome to be achieved is exceedingly poor. These same traditions also provide ethical guidance about physicians' responsibilities under futile circumstances. Thus, for example, the well-known Hippocratic oath identifies the tasks of physicians as twofold: first, to "use treatment to help the sick according to my ability and judgment"; second, "never [to use treatment] with a view to injury and wrongdoing."[9] The oath provides a basis, therefore, for claiming that physicians not only should *be permitted* to refrain from using futile interventions but also should be *encouraged* or *required* to refrain from using futile treatments because such interventions fall outside the scope of helping the sick. Also, they cause "injury and wrongdoing" because they raise false hope, inflict unnecessary pain, prolong suffering, make the dying process less humane and dignified, and most of all, distract physicians from providing palliation and comfort.

The Platonic tradition gives similar guidance. Medicine is a good so long as "the patient is freed from a great evil, so that it is profitable to submit to the pain and recover health."[10] But a medical regimen is not a pleasant thing; patients do not enjoy it. Plato cautioned that physicians cannot determine whether burdens are offset by benefits by focusing narrowly on specific pathological problems. Instead, the physician must take stock of the whole patient while recognizing that "the part can never be well unless the whole is well." Thus, Plato condemned the physicians of Hellas for "disregarding the whole," and added, "You ought not to attempt to cure the eyes without the head, or the head without the body . . . [or] the body without the soul."[11] Bringing nutrients to the stomach or breath to the lungs does not necessarily benefit the patient or restore health. Rather, to heal the patient literally means (according to the *Oxford English Dictionary*) "to make whole or sound in bodily condition." What then should the physician do when wholeness cannot be achieved? What is the physician's ethical duty?

Just as the ancient Greek physician was instructed to do good and avoid harming the patient, so too, the colonial physician was supposed to be an honorable person who could be relied on to make the patient's good paramount. The eighteenth-century physician belonged to a profession that espoused caring for the sick and protecting the public's welfare. In some accounts, beneficence is a value built into the very reality of medicine as a special kind of human activity—namely, an activity of responding to the need of sick persons for care, cure, help, and healing.[12]

Today, the profession remains committed to accomplishing certain moral ends, such as

1. reassuring the worried well who have no disease or injury;
2. diagnosing disease or injury;
3. helping the patient to understand the disease;
4. preventing disease or injury;
5. curing the disease or repairing the injury;
6. lessening the pain or disability caused by disease or injury;

7. helping the patient to live with pain or disability;
8. helping the patient die with dignity and peace.[13]

Medically futile interventions not only fail to achieve these aims, but also frustrate efforts to do so. Thus, futile interventions also frustrate efforts to help the patient understand the disease, its prognosis, and its effects on the patient's life (end no. 3); increase, rather than lessen, the pain caused by the disease (6); and stand in the way of helping the patient die with dignity and peace (8).

While other values, such as autonomy, are now recognized as integral to the physician's ethical role, physicians do not see their goal as simply doing whatever the patient wishes. Instead, physicians continue to affirm a duty to help patients.

The Weakest Ethical Stance: Physicians Should Be Permitted to Refrain from Offering Futile Treatment

A central aim of the profession of medicine is to use the art and science of medicine for the purpose of *helping* the sick. But futile treatment, by definition, is superfluous to helping the patient. In Mr. Tanney's case, the overwhelming odds were that CPR efforts would not benefit him. It follows then that physicians who refrained from CPR, rather than attempting resuscitation, would in no way be remiss in their duty to help the patient (the duty of beneficence).

We emphasize that the primary obligation of doctors and nurses is to benefit patients. Expressed differently, the subject of medical care is the suffering patient, not a failing organ system or body part. Thus, even when interventions can produce physiological *effects* or prolong *biological life*, they may not confer a benefit that the patient can appreciate. In these instances, the requirement of beneficence does not apply and treatment is not ethically obligatory. Often, where futile treatments provide a psychological benefit, such benefits can be achieved in other, and better, ways.

It follows that patients who demand nonbeneficial medical treatments from their physicians hold an exaggerated idea of the duties required of physicians. Moreover, physicians who offer futile interventions are not advocating for patients, but are instead deceiving patients and compromising professional standards. By offering a treatment to a patient or family, a physician conveys that the treatment represents a medically acceptable alternative. But if the treatment is almost certain to fail and the patient is misled into believing in the treatment's efficacy, then the physician has violated the patient's trust. If the physician informs the patient that the treatment is futile and offers it anyway, a confusing double message is thereby conveyed.

The provision of futile treatment is additionally objectionable because physicians (and other health professionals) are obligated to uphold professional standards of care. The idea here is that medicine, nursing, and the other healing professions are not practiced *merely on demand*, but instead aspire to *moral goals*, such as *helping* the sick. Not only does the physician let down the patient, the physician lets down every other member of the medical profession. When physicians prescribe treatments that they are reasonably certain will not improve a patient's condition, they degrade the practice of medicine. They ally medicine with quackery and charlatanism.

Finally, the use of futile measures is ethically objectionable in situations where it runs contrary to the physician's personal moral standards. In this case, a refusal to allow the physician to withhold or withdraw futile interventions does not take seriously the physician's own sense of personal moral integrity. It would be akin to forcing physicians who oppose abortions to perform them. In these cases, requiring the use of futile interventions wrongly signals that physicians are merely tools for enacting others' (patients', institutions') nonmedical goals, rather than individuals and members of a profession who possess independent ethical standards and ends. Thus, we would conclude that at a very minimum physicians are *ethically permitted* to refrain from offering futile treatment.

A Moderate Ethical Stance: Physicians Should Be Encouraged to Refrain from Offering Futile Therapies

Suppose that we agree that Dr. Sylvester cannot be compelled to attempt CPR on Mr. Tanney. Dr. Sylvester would reasonably conclude, therefore, that he was free either to *use* the futile treatment or to *withhold* it. Either way, his actions would be above reproach.

Some patients and families cling to faith in the miraculous powers of medicine that far exceed medicine's actual scientific capabilities; some hold that they are entitled to their hopes and that medicine is duty-bound to serve them. The difficulty with this claim is that shocking the heart with high-voltage electricity or pounding on Mr. Tanney's chest in a futile attempt to get the heart started is not an ethically neutral act. Harm is inevitable: ribs can be broken, the trachea damaged by hasty efforts at intubation. Not uncommonly, the brain never completely recovers from oxygen deprivation. In fact, cardiac arrest is the third leading cause of coma, second only to trauma and drug overdose.[14] Most hospitalized patients who undergo attempts at CPR—even those treated with induced hypothermia—never survive to leave the hospital, and some of those who do sustain significant neurological impairment.[15]

These harms would be justified only if they were matched by compensatory benefits. But the benefit realized by Mr. Tanney would be only a false hope that he would somehow pull through, that a miracle would happen. The truth is that even if Mr. Tanney had survived the cardiac arrest and retained consciousness, he would only return to the discomfort and suffering associated with his metastatic cancer and almost certainly would never survive to hospital discharge. This violates the first ethic of the medical profession: Do no harm (nonmaleficence). Futile interventions often increase patients' suffering and discomfort. Thus, the ethical principle of doing no harm will sometimes support a positive duty to refrain from futile interventions.

Even when futile interventions do not exact such a heavy toll, we would argue that physicians should be *encouraged* to withhold and withdraw them because medicine's goal has always been to help the patient, and futile interventions fail to do so. Rather, medicine's aim has always been to help the sick. Affirming this age-old ethic, the President's Commission for the Study of Ethical Problems in Medicine and Biomedical and Behavioral Research stated in 1983 that "the care available from health care professionals is generally limited to what is consistent with role-related professional standards and conscientiously held personal beliefs."[16]

How appropriate is it for medicine to be the only profession with unlimited obligations to the people it serves? Would those who claim that patients and families can demand anything they want from doctors lay similar claims on other professions? Not at all. Let us look, for example, at the legal profession. A person accused of murder deserves a full and vigorous defense by his attorney. Does that mean that after conviction and life sentence, the permanently incarcerated prisoner can demand that the attorney phone the governor every day in search of a miraculous change of mind and clemency? Surely at some point the lawyer would declare a limit to her professional obligations to the client. A client who orders an architect to design a beautiful but structurally unsound building made of glass would learn that architects are limited by building codes as well as by the codes of their profession. Similarly, physicians are not and never have been obligated to do anything a patient wants, such as treating in expectation of a miracle. Medical treatment is not simply a consumer good to be bought and sold.

Finally, there is an even more important reason why physicians should avoid pursuing futile life-saving treatments: because the obsessive pursuit of such treatments often causes them to neglect a whole other set of duties—relieving pain and responding to the dying patient's situation in an empathic and caring way. Attention spent on debating useless interventions often distracts physicians from these goals. Indeed, we have found that all too often the medical team is consumed in heated debate over whether or not to attempt aggressive technological interventions, meanwhile falling sadly short in their responsibility to meet the patient's physical, emotional, and spiritual needs. At the end of life, the physician's primary focus should be on helping the patient achieve as good a death as possible. We emphasize that, in conversations with patients and families, providers should be careful to distinguish between the withholding of futile interventions on the one hand, and the provision of comfort and care on the other. Rather than saying to the patient (or loved one), "There is nothing I can do for you," health professionals should instead affirm that *everything possible* will be done to ensure the patient's comfort and dignity.

As we discussed in Chapter 1, futility comes from the word *futtlis*, meaning "leaky." Traditionally, *futtilis* referred to a religious vessel that was wide at the top and extremely narrow at the bottom. The futtilis was used in religious ceremonies, where the idea was to fill it, and then let it tip over. Because of its shape, it was impossible to keep liquid in it for any length of time. And so, in a sense, it became futile to attempt to preserve any contents in it.

Recalling this derivation is useful because it reminds us that many of the futile gestures that we make in medicine actually carry symbolic (ritual) connotations. Sometimes, when we are trying to express love, affection, respect, and honor for a departing loved one, we insist on going through futile gestures—CPR, ventilator, intensive care unit, tube feedings. It is important for all of us to recognize that there are better ways, both substantively and symbolically, for us to honor a person than to cause all sorts of harmful interruptions in the dying process.

A Strong Ethical Stance: Physicians Should Be Required to Refrain from Offering Futile Interventions

So far we have defended two progressively stronger claims concerning the ethical responsibilities of physicians in futile circumstances. The weak claim asserts that physicians are free to withhold or cease futile therapies. The moderate stance maintains that physicians should be encouraged to do so. We now make the stronger case that the ethical *obligation* of physicians is to *forgo* futile interventions.

The bases for this stronger claim are fourfold. First, in the absence of a general professional ethic affirming the scope and limits of physicians' obligations, the meaning and ethical implications of futility are vulnerable to abuse. For example, if Dr. Garland and Dr. Sylvester were free to use "futility" to mean whatever they wished, then their debate over whether to attempt CPR on Mr. Tanney might have had many possible hidden subtexts. Did Dr. Garland think Mr. Tanney too old to be receiving such expensive medical care? Was she subconsciously withholding CPR because the patient was not as pleasant, as interesting, or as grateful as other patients in her care? Perhaps Dr. Sylvester did not experience this, having known Mr. Tanney only briefly. Did Dr. Garland find her time taken away from other patients whom she thought had more need for her and better chances of a successful outcome? All these could lead to the term "futility" being invoked in a variety of subterfuges for rationing, cost containment, or refusals to treat certain categories of patients—HIV-infected, mentally or physically disabled, or elderly individuals.

In other words, the absence of a profession-wide standard governing the ethical responsibilities of physicians under futile circumstances invites abuse by allowing physicians to act according to their own (subconscious or deliberately concealed) arbitrary goals. To avoid such abuse, the profession of medicine must affirm a clear and consistent definition of futility and set systematic standards for its members. Only then can misuses of the term be recognized for what they are. Only then can patients be assured that their wishes and best interests will not be subordinated to inappropriate economic and social considerations.

A second reason for ethically requiring physicians to refrain from futile treatment is that the public rightly looks to the practitioners of medicine to set standards for appropriate medical treatment. Physicians in our society practice medicine as part of a publicly sanctioned profession: society grants the profession authority to certify individual practitioners as competent to act in the best interests of patients. By virtue of receiving such authority, the profession receives the public's trust, just as other professions receive the right and responsibility to provide legal counsel, maintain accounting records, design bridges, and educate. To be worthy of this trust, a profession is obliged to set ethical guidelines for its practitioners. The medical profession abdicates its responsibility to society if it leaves the setting of standards for beneficial and nonbeneficial medical practice to individual clinicians.

Third, as we noted in Chapter 5, futile interventions expend finite resources. Considerations of justice thus lend support to the claim that physicians should not be offering useless treatments to patients. For even when the resources in question are plentiful, the dollars to pay for health care are always finite and scarce. This is owing to the fact that there are other things besides health care that we as a society choose to spend money on. And even within the area of health care itself, is it fair to devote scarce resources to ventilator support or tube feeding of an individual who will never regain consciousness while refusing to pay for basic health care for the poor and uninsured? These questions are the context in which futility decisions are made. For reasons of justice, physicians should not be using futile interventions.

Finally, physicians are ethically obligated to avoid futile medicine because its use exploits the public's fears and feeds inflated ideas about what medicine can achieve. Today not only do Americans fear death, but also those many thousands who made an instant bestseller out of a how-to-commit-suicide book published by the Hemlock Society seem to fear *medicine* as an unrestrained force lacking humanity and common sense.[17] Contemporary physicians—even more than did ancient physicians—bear special obligations in this regard because they practice in a society that extols, even worships, technology and clings tenaciously to exaggerated beliefs about what medicine can accomplish. To counter this tendency, the profession of medicine should take a firm and public stand stating the limits of what their profession can and will do. In the absence of such a commitment, individuals and families and society will continue to hold physicians and hospitals hostage by insisting that medicine owes them miraculous feats. Or, they will make rash end-of-life decisions out of distrust for the medical profession, thus depriving themselves of the wide variety of beneficial treatments and care that can be offered.

Professional medical and biomedical ethical organizations are clearly rising to the challenge and affirming medicine's limits. During the 1980s and 1990s, professional medical bioethics associations began taking formal positions and recommending that futile treatments be withheld, or be withdrawn if already under way. As early as 1983, the President's Commission for the Study of Ethical Problems in Medicine and Biomedical and Behavioral Research declared: "A health care professional has an obligation to allow a patient to choose from among medically acceptable treatment options . . . or to reject all options. No one, however, has an obligation to provide interventions that would, in his or her judgment, be countertherapeutic."[18] Subsequent statements explicitly recognize the term "futility" and caution physicians against applying futile interventions. In 1987, the Hastings Center, an internationally recognized bioethics organization, stated in its *Guidelines on the Termination of Life-Sustaining Treatment and the Care of the Dying* that "if a treatment is clearly futile . . . there is no obligation to provide the treatment."[19]

Other respected medical organizations followed suit. In 1991, the American Medical Association's Council on Ethical and Judicial Affairs published "Guidelines for the Appropriate Use of Do-Not-Resuscitate Orders." The council held that CPR efforts may be withheld, even if previously requested by the patient, "when efforts to resuscitate a patient are judged by the treating physician to be futile." In the same year, the American Thoracic Society (an organization of the American Lung Association) took a similar stand, saying that "forcing physicians to provide medical interventions that are clearly futile would undermine the ethical integrity of the medical profession." During the same period, the Society of Critical Care Medicine's Task Force on Ethics published a consensus report stating that "treatments that offer no benefit and serve to prolong the dying process should not be employed." In 1993, the Ethics Committee of the Society of Critical Care Medicine specified patients with severe, irreversible brain damage, irreversible multiple-organ failure, and metastatic cancer unresponsive to treatment as categories of "patients who *may* be excluded from the ICU, whether beds are available or not." The committee also designated those who refuse intensive care, who are brain-dead, or who are in a permanent vegetative state as "patients who *should* be excluded." And most recently, in 2009, the American Medical Association expanded on its earlier declaration by seeking congressional legislation "that will allow the creation of a methodology directed by physicians (MDs/DOs) that permits physicians (MDs/DOs) to either not engage in or to suspend futile care at the end of life," and asked that physicians be legally protected from liability when "such decisions are made in good faith and within the standard of care with clear and convincing legal and ethical standards."[20]

Objections and Responses

Having set forth a compelling argument to show that physicians are obligated to help patients, and should not use futile medical treatments, we now summarize a series of objections from the literature, which we have discussed in more detail elsewhere.[21]

Why shouldn't the patient, rather than the doctor, always be allowed to decide what to do when treatment is futile? In other words, why should futile treatment not be offered to the patient as an option?

Geriatrician Thomas Finucane posed this question in the form of a thought experiment: "If you were to suddenly die now and the probability of surviving with attempted treatment were 1 in 100, would you accept the attempt? Now let us stipulate that the attempt would be free and painless and would, if successful, return you to your current level of function. I would answer 'yes,' promptly. I would answer 'yes' at 1 in 1000. I wouldn't consider the chance to be 'negligible' nor the attempt to be 'inappropriate' in a general sense."[22]

Sure. And if we all had wings, we could fly. The problem with formulating the question this way is that in the real world, life-saving medical treatments are never free and painless. Rather, they are by nature invasive, burdensome, and fraught with serious, lingering harms. That is why physicians are expected to use their powers not at will but with care and restraint. Of course, there is a procedure that meets the criteria of being free, painless, rarely successful, but reputedly now and then miraculous. It is called prayer. The question then becomes: If the patient feels entitled to it, is the *physician* obligated to perform it? We have already argued that physicians are not obligated to offer treatments that are so likely to fail that any success would be considered a miracle. Physicians can offer only what nature allows and cannot accept responsibility for being something they are not—miracle workers. And so, we maintain, physicians are limited in their duty to patients by a common-sense notion of quantitative futility.

We also offer the following analogical argument in support of quantitative futility. This argument begins by drawing an analogy between futile treatments and placebos. Placebos (from the word meaning "to please") are medications that display no objective specific activity for the condition being treated. In drug trials involving control subjects, placebos are usually capsules with a small amount of an inert substance like lactose. They are necessary for comparison because the "placebo effect" of a drug, which is perceived as a physiological or psychological benefit and which operates through a psychological mechanism, can be as high as 30 percent or even higher.[23] A dramatic illustration of the placebo effect occurred during World War II when a military pharmacy ran out of narcotics. To the physicians' astonishment, soldiers with severe war injuries, who were not told they were receiving only sterile saline injections, experienced pain relief. What can we conclude from this experience? Even in the case of severe pain, sterile saline might conceivably work. If physicians were morally obligated to offer any treatment that might make a patient feel good or that might conceivably make a patient feel good, the physician would be *obligated,* in the absence of a proven treatment, to offer this placebo. But physicians are *not* morally obligated to offer a placebo when no treatment is available, for good reasons. Any trust between doctor and patient—not to mention the psychological benefits of all medicines—would be destroyed if patients knew that physicians prescribed medicines whether or not they believed in their therapeutic efficacy. Patients would rightly be concerned not only about therapeutic efficacy but also about therapeutic deception.

But what about qualitative futility? Why shouldn't patients be allowed to decide for themselves the qualities of life they would find acceptable?

We believe a distinction is in order. Some qualitatively poor results should indeed be the patient's prerogative. However, other sorts of qualitatively poor results fall clearly outside the range of medical goals and need not be offered as options. The clearest of these qualitatively poor results is continued biological life without consciousness. The patient has no right to demand of medicine to be sustained in a state in which he or she has no capacity to appreciate the life prolonged by treatment and no purpose other than mere vegetative survival. The physician should not offer this option or services to achieve it. Other qualitatively poor results include survival that requires the constant monitoring and ventilatory support of the intensive care unit or an acute care hospital—measures which effectively prevent the patient from achieving any other life goals, including participation in the human community. Admittedly, seriously ill patients fall along a continuum, and there are well-known examples of the most remarkable achievements of life goals despite the most burdensome disabilities (the wheelchair-bound—but *not* hospital bound—theoretical physicist Stephen Hawking comes to mind). However, if survival requires the patient's entire *preoccupation* with intensive medical treatment, to the extent that the patient cannot achieve any other life goals (thus obviating the goal of medical care), the treatment is producing an effect but not a benefit. It should not be offered to the patient, and the patient's family has no right to demand it.

Specifically excluded from our account is medical treatment for people for whom such treatment offers the opportunity to achieve life goals, however limited. For example, the French magazine editor Jean-Dominique Bauby had a stroke and was left in a locked-in syndrome, completely paralyzed except for his ability to blink his left eyelid to indicate "yes" or "no." With the help of a transcriber, who over a period of 10 months repeatedly recited letters, the blinking Bauby was able to compose a remarkable book, *The Diving Bell and the Butterfly*, before he died of pneumonia. Thus, people whose illnesses are severe enough to require frequent hospitalization, residents of nursing homes, or people who have severe physical or mental disabilities are not, in themselves, objects of futile treatments. We wish to emphasize: such people (or their surrogates) have the right to receive or reject any medical treatment according to their own perception of benefit compared with burdens. We also suggest that the medical profession respond to our futility proposal not by eagerly seeking to give up on severely compromised patients but by looking for better ways to support patients *outside* the acute care setting (like that received by Bauby)—in skilled nursing facilities and even at home—where patients can sometimes have more interactions with loved ones, friends, and the community at large.

We conclude that the ethical requirement to respect patient autonomy, which motivates this objection, is overstated. While respect for autonomy certainly gives patients a negative right not to be interfered with, it does not give them a right to coerce others (the medical profession) to provide them with whatever medical means they want. Nor is autonomy a value that stands alone. Instead it must be considered together with other values, such as doing good, avoiding harm, and justice.

Won't preventing patients from making their own assessment of qualitative futility lead to abuse, neglect, and a retreat to the paternalistic "silent world"[24] of the past in which doctors avoided communication with their patients? Because the doctor-patient relationship is inherently unequal, with physicians exerting greater power and authority than patients, doesn't granting physicians authority to limit futile treatment only exacerbate this power differential and grant physicians excessive power and authority?

Related to the concern about the physician's power is the concern that physicians will abuse their power and authority. We acknowledge that the potential for abuse is present. We would deplore the use of our proposal to excuse doctors from engaging patients in ongoing informed dialogue. But by holding physicians to openly declared standards of medical futility, our proposal not only authorizes physicians to exercise professional judgment and develop empirically based standards of care, but also limits their power and prevents its arbitrary exercise. And we must point out that the alternative—allowing patients or families unlimited choices—is also subject to abuse, for example, when patients and surrogates intimidate hospitals into providing extravagant, nonbeneficial treatments by threatening to sensationalize their case in the media.[25]

If futility is a value judgment, doesn't it follow that physicians are no better equipped than lay people to render this judgment?

We agree that physicians could never claim authority to render futility judgments under the guise of some purely objective and value-free "scientific" or "technical" expertise. Instead, the proper basis for assigning physicians authority to set standards for the practice of medicine is that an ethical dimension is an integral component of the historical and contemporary role of the profession in society. In the first edition of *Wrong Medicine*, we quoted the philosopher and medical ethicist Margaret Battin, who said that even when the patient gives informed consent to treatment, "it is the physician who identifies the problem, frames any suggested solution to it, and controls how many alternative solutions are proposed."[26] This is only partly true today. In the 15 years since the publication of the first edition of *Wrong Medicine*, an entirely new source of medical information has become available—the Internet. In 1995 the Internet was accessed by fewer than 5 percent of Americans; now that number is almost 80 percent.

Unfortunately, many Web sites that purport to offer medical advice are unreliable; patients should be careful to discuss their claims with a physician. At its best, this source of medical information grants the patient a supplementary pathway "to explore whether the problem could be seen in some other way or as some different sort of problem, whether other sorts of solutions could be proposed, whether in making the choice to give or withhold consent the patient is making a choice among all the reasonable alternatives, and, sometimes, whether there is really any problem at all."[27] Likewise, direct consumer marketing of prescription drugs and other medical treatments can inform patients about options, but these should always be discussed with physicians or others competent to give advice to individual patients.

Even with all the avenues of information now open to consumers of medical care, physicians still wield enormous power in modern society in almost every conceivable circumstance, and for this reason society rightly expects them to show restraint and to practice their craft in an ethical way. The fact that society deplores those who practice medicine solely to make a profit, achieve status, or selfishly exploit their power, reveals that we hold physicians to a high moral standard and expect them to use their skills to help sick people and promote the good of society. This expectation will continue to be justified only so long as the profession of medicine espouses and practices according to ideals of service and advocacy for patients.

We reiterate the point that physicians are obligated to make *medical* decisions—namely, decisions aimed at healing the suffering patient. Merely preserving biological existence is not a medical goal. Vitalist notions that a permanently unconscious body or a dead body whose heart and lungs are being kept active by mechanical means—that these conditions must be prolonged—are not medical concepts. And although some members of society may hold such imperatives as deeply felt beliefs, those beliefs cannot be imposed on health professionals any more than a deep belief in the importance of teaching creationism can be imposed on the educational profession.

Won't requiring physicians to refrain from using futile treatments unfairly violate the religious convictions of some patients, and even of some doctors and nurses?

This is an important question, because most persons in this country—including patients and health professionals—either observe or are significantly influenced by religious beliefs. Nurses are peculiarly vulnerable in these situations. Following their own religious beliefs, patients can demand and refuse treatments, and physicians can order and refuse to order them. But nurses by the nature of their intermediary role in the medical hierarchy—obligated to both parties—are often locked in the middle of painful conflicts. Their power to control events, not to mention their own actions, is severely limited, and their sense of job security often threatened. Indeed, some of the most difficult ethical consultations we have conducted deal with the so-called "moral stresses" of nurses forced to carry out orders that they feel are harmful and inappropriate.

However, as the theologian James W. Walters points out, while religion offers "fundamental perspectives which inform society's dilemmas," it must, like other forces in society, "make a public case for its views."[28] And contrary to the notion of a single immutable theology, in fact all religious traditions have undergone reexamination and reinterpretation throughout history, even within the Catholic Church, which is traditionally regarded as representing timeless, unchanging views. Catholic scholar and jurist John T. Noonan Jr. writes:

> Wide shifts in the teaching of moral duties, once presented as part of Christian doctrine by the magisterium, have occurred. In each case one can see the displacement of a principle or principles that had been taken as dispositive—in the case of usury, that a loan confers no right to profit; in the case of marriage, that all marriages are indissoluble; in the case of slavery, that war gives a right to enslave and that ownership of a slave gives title to the slave's offspring; in the case of religious liberty, that error has no rights and the fidelity to the Christian faith may be physically enforced. . . . In the course of this displacement of one set of principles, what was forbidden became lawful (the cases of usury and marriage); what was permissible became unlawful (the case of slavery); and what was required became forbidden (the persecution of heretics).[29]

Professor Charles Curran also objects to a Roman Catholic theology that presents itself as immutable, eternal, and unchanging, rather than emphasizing "evolution, growth, change and historicity."[30] And the Catholic theologian Richard McBrien of Notre Dame agrees that "there are many different approaches to theological issues." These approaches are inevitably influenced by historical context and evolving contingencies that require repeated interpretations with respect to the specific application of religious principles to the ever-changing complexities of modern medicine. "All the principles that the church lives by," McBrien declares, "are principles that come out of its own experience."[31]

In the past, Bible-quoting religious leaders used religious principles to justify slavery and suppression of women, to name just two examples of values almost universally rejected today by mainstream American theologians and the wider society. It is particularly important to keep this in mind with regard to the medical context. Both the Jewish and Christian traditions make the claim that life is of supreme value, a gift of God to be held in trust. But what exactly is meant by life? Biological existence? Cells possessing human chromosomes? Personhood? As we have already noted, modern medical technology has created many states of life between health and death that were unimaginable in the days when the major religions evolved.

In the best of circumstances, physicians and members of the clergy pool their skills and knowledge to help patients come to terms with their situation. Sometimes hospital chaplains can play a particularly valuable and comforting role by correcting a devout family's misapprehensions about what is ordained in their religion. For example, Catholicism does *not* absolutely forbid the use of pain medications that might accelerate death, nor forbid the withdrawal of life support under any circumstances. In fact, under the principle of "double effect," it is Catholic theology that has provided the most cogent moral guidance in the first instance, namely, that as long as the physician's intent is to achieve a good (alleviating suffering), then an unavoidable side-effect (increasing the risk of death) is not deemed sinful, provided the good effect is sufficient to outweigh the unintended bad effect. In the second instance, Catholicism does not require physicians to impose on their patients "extraordinary" treatments, namely, interventions that are capable of achieving little or no benefit or whose burdens outweigh any benefits.

One example of a thoughtful and knowledgeable interpretation of essential religious values in the light of modern medical technology is provided by the Christian physician James Reitman,[32] citing Ecclesiastes 9:3–6 (New International Version):

> This is the evil in everything that happens under the sun: The same destiny overtakes all. The hearts of men, moreover, are full of evil and there is madness in their hearts while they live, and afterward they join the dead. Anyone who is among the living has hope—even a live dog is better off than a dead lion!

> For the living know that they will die,
>> but the dead know nothing;
>> they have no further reward,
>> and even the memory of them is forgotten.
> Their love, their hate
>> and their jealousy have long since vanished;
>> never again will they have a part
>> in anything that happens under the sun.

Reitman found in these biblical lines the fundamental wisdom that death is impartial and inevitable for all, and that human beings have impure motivations and lack insight. Nevertheless, the passage points out, life has meaning (which justifies hope), regardless of a person's status, as long as life exists. But what gives meaning to life is the exercise of awareness ("For the living *know* that they will die"); emotive responsivity ("Their love, their hate and their jealousy"); and volitional capacity (having "a part in anything that happens under the sun"). Reitman argues that as the capacity for any or all of these qualities erodes with illness and suffering, there is a progressive decrease in the potential for meaning and hope. Physicians should always take this eroding potential into account in making medical decisions, including whether to provide aggressive life support or to withhold such treatments on grounds of futility. The duty of the physician, he states, is not to err in either direction, "*either* of usurping the prerogative of a sovereign God over life [as defined in Ecclesiastes] *or* of prematurely removing hope."[33]

With regard to medical treatments, Catholic moralists have long distinguished between ordinary (obligatory) and extraordinary (nonobligatory) measures. In the Catholic tradition, neither futile or nonbeneficial treatments nor extremely burdensome treatments are held to be obligatory. Thus, although preservation of life is regarded as a value requiring ordinary efforts, it is not a paramount or overriding value requiring extraordinary efforts.

In the Jewish tradition, the commentary of the fourteenth-century Provençal Halakhist R. Menachem ha-Meiri is often cited today as one of the authorities for the mandate to pursue maximal efforts at life preservation: "Even if [a person found alive under a fallen house] cannot live more than an hour, in that hour he may repent and utter the confession."[34] Clearly, the commentary emerged from a time when human biological existence and personhood were experienced as coterminous, with consciousness typically ending only a short time before death. Such reasoning did not anticipate or take into account the impossibility of confession during the decades of unconsciousness possible in a patient preserved by modern technology in the permanent vegetative state. As the contemporary Jewish theologian Rabbi Immanuel Jakobovits points out, all the authoritative Jewish sources "refer to an individual in whom death is expected to be imminent, three days or less in rabbinic references."[35] It is also interesting to note that rabbinical distinctions were made between acts viewed as hastening death, such as closing the eyes of the dying person, and acts considered "impediments to death," such as the noise made by a nearby woodchopper or salt placed on the tongue. Thus, though they come from a historical context that no longer exists, these theological pronouncements nevertheless resonate with our own modern debate about the use of technologies and food and fluids that "prolong dying." Dr. Fred Rosner, Rabbi J. David Bleich, and Rabbi Dr. Menachem M. Brayer ask, "Who can make the fine distinction between prolonging life and prolonging the act of dying? The former comes within the physician's reference, the latter does not."[36] Indeed, the sources for Jewish ethics—the Talmud, the Torah, and rabbinical commentaries—reveal a rich history of interpretation in each era and society, activities that continue today.[37] As the Catholic scholar John Noonan summarizes, "In new conditions, with new insight, an old rule need not be preserved in order to honor a past discipline."[38]

It should be evident, therefore, that medicine cannot assume that religion imposes fixed and detailed rules on what constitutes futile treatment and whether or not to attempt such treatments. Furthermore, in American society, the separation of church and state both protects religious diversity and restrains any group from imposing a single theological interpretation on public policy formation. Under the U.S. Constitution, every citizen is free to hold any religious conviction, but the state is not permitted to impose that conviction on other individuals or on society in general. Similarly, standards of medical treatment cannot reflect the religious creed of any single group, but instead should represent the outcome of open and reasoned debate encompassing a wide range of religious and other values. Only in this manner does the profession receive the sanction of the entire society that it is called on to serve. And although particular individuals and groups in the United States can always be expected to make claims on medicine that are based on religious and other grounds, the profession of medicine is rightly governed by values and standards that are its own. In the interest of religious pluralism and of preventing the imposition of religious beliefs on others, the United States has allowed those with specific religious convictions to form their own health care systems. One example is Catholic hospitals, which do not perform abortions. In like manner, religious groups who demand medical treatments outside the mainstream of American society, such as unlimited life-support for patients in permanent vegetative state, could develop their own health care facilities devoted to treating members who share this belief.[39]

Won't granting the medical profession authority to define medical futility and set ethical standards start us down a perilous and slippery slope, returning us to the unhappy days of physician paternalism or, worse, to a society and medical profes-

sion that contributed to the horrors of the Nazi era? How can we be assured that physicians won't apply racial and other invidious stereotypes when evaluating patients' quality of life? How can we be confident that physicians won't extend their authority from extreme cases, in which interventions are clearly futile, to other kinds of cases where the quality of life associated with an intervention is impaired, but remains well worth living?

We do not dismiss such concerns lightly. The abuse of futility can produce devastating consequences, and physicians are not immune from the prejudices and stereotypes legion in the larger society. Nonetheless, we reiterate that the most effective way to stem possible abuses is to make explicit and publicly accountable policies regarding the definition and ethical implications of medical futility. Most important, and a crucial distinction from the attitudes of the Nazi era, decisions about medical futility must be patient-centered and not grounded in a singular ideology or notion of societal good. And to those who fear the potential abuses of medical futility we must sadly report our everyday experiences. Today, every day, at the bedside, futility judgments are being made in a variety of inconsistent ways. And the physicians making these judgments are not accountable to their colleagues or to the public, nor are their judgments measured against specific and openly declared professional standards. By demanding that physicians be held to such standards, we actually *limit* the power of physicians to impose their will.

A related charge is that talk about futility is in reality nothing more than a convenient code for talking about rationing and cost containment. If that is the case, isn't it manipulative and unethical to disguise economic matters in this fashion?

We respond by reiterating that rationing, cost containment, and futility convey very different meanings and ethical implications. That is why it is essential for us to address these issues openly. Failure to do so will continue the confusion and emotional distortions that have made sensible discourse so difficult and so susceptible to political posturing. Futility refers to a specific treatment-benefit relationship in a particular patient. Futility means that a treatment offers no reasonable benefit to that patient—whether or not it is cheap or easily available. By contrast, rationing refers to treatments that *do* offer benefits but that cannot be offered because they are too costly or scarce or because other patients are assigned priority. Cost containment also differs in its meaning and ethical implications from futility because the goal of cost containment is to reduce overall medical expenditures.

Sometimes, as we have already pointed out, the question of providing medical treatment is posed in terms of economics alone. "If I am rich," the question may go, "and can afford to pay for years of intensive medical treatment for my child's permanent vegetative state, why can't I have it?" Our answer is: "Because you really *can't* afford to pay for it. The cost is not merely the room rate of the ICU and the various supplies and professional fees, but rather, involves a fraction of a far more vast sum of money (taken from taxing others), including that expended on constructing the hospital facilities, on developing the treatments, on training all the people who have provided every aspect of health care, and on the research and training of all those who trained them, and so on. But most of all, you can't pay for the health care taken away from others while it is being provided for your child." So our response to those who call for the freedom to have any medical care they want is that in the process of U.S. health care reform, our democratic society first must provide a "decent minimum" that is satisfactory to the society as a whole. Beyond that decent minimum our society will certainly allow "buy-ups" for those who wish to seek additional medical goals, such as cosmetic surgery, perhaps. But it does not therefore follow that persons will be entitled to buy *anything* they want from health providers, even treatments that serve no medical goal.

Life is always better than death. Thus, no matter how poor the quality of life becomes, it is always preferable to having no life at all. The idea of "qualitative futility" that we submit is thus unpersuasive. Death, according to this objection, is the greatest evil.

In response we point out that death is not itself an experience of any sort. After all, there is no subject that survives death who can have experience in the sense that we usually understand this. Once a person dies (i.e., has total and irreversible cessation of brain function, as defined in the law), or, even short of this, when there is no higher brain function, it is not physically possible for an individual to have conscious experience because the part of the brain responsible for experience is destroyed.

Philosophers have long argued that our tendency to fear death, and to regard it as the greatest evil possible, is not only unsupported but also irrational. Thus, the ancient Greek philosopher Lucretius argued that it is irrational to think death is bad for us because we do not think the nonexistence preceding our births is bad for us. According to Lucretius, when we compare this period of nonexistence with death, we see the two are mirror images, alike in all respects. The argument, sometimes referred to as the asymmetry argument, can be stated as follows.[40]

1. Being dead is a state of nonexistence.
2. Being not yet conceived is a state of nonexistence.
3. We are not disturbed by our past nonexistence.
4. Therefore, it is inconsistent and irrational to be disturbed by our future nonexistence.

Thus understood, death is neither good nor evil, but instead a neutral state.

If this argument is persuasive and death is indeed a neutral state, why then do we fear death? It is almost a cliché to say that "people fear dying, not death." In other words, we fear that the dying process that precedes death may be painful and prolonged. We worry about the loss of control that can accompany the ravages of disease.

But it is not only dying, but also death itself, that people (irrationally) fear. People would not be so concerned about dying if it were not followed by death. The conclusion of the asymmetry argument presents a paradox: a puzzling conclusion we seem driven to by our reasoning, but one which is highly counterintuitive. Intuitively, most of us fear death and will take every measure to avoid it. While our fear of death can be adaptive in many instances (even if irrational)—for example, by helping us to make good lifestyle choices or avoid excessive risks—for a dying patient the desire to avoid death or the tendency to regard it as the ultimate evil is neither rational nor adaptive. In this context, the view that death is the greatest evil leads to tragic choices.

Our Ethical Imperative

Even if we cannot banish our irrational fear of death, we can perhaps stop fighting death at the end of life when death is inevitable. We can find better and wiser ways to cope with our fear. In ancient Greek society, death was regarded much more as an accepted part of life. According to Greek mythology, the Fates appear three nights after a child's birth to determine the course of its life. They are often depicted as old crones or hags who are cold and unfeeling. They control the metaphorical thread of life of every person: Clotho spins the thread of life from her staff onto her spindle, Lachesis measures the thread of life allotted to each person with her measuring rod, and Atropos is the cutter of the thread of life. When she cuts the thread with her shears, someone on Earth dies.

While we are not fatalists in the classical sense, we believe there is much wisdom in the story of the Fates. In modern times, the inevitability of death is something that we must humbly acknowledge as the Greeks did. We must give up many of our modern myths, which depict the doctor as God-like or capable of performing miracles. We must humbly accept when the limits of medicine and science are reached. Rather than holding out as heroic aggressive efforts to beat all odds and vanquish death, we must sometimes see the ability to stop as heroic and hold in high regard the importance of being with and caring for the patient.

We conclude that physicians should generally be required to refrain from using futile interventions. This general ethical stance should be publicly endorsed by the medical profession, embodied in institutional policies, and presented clearly and frankly to the public. Such a stance should include a candid acknowledgment that doctors should not arrogantly offer, nor should patients unreasonably demand, unlimited treatments. This stance forces us to reexamine the doctor-patient relationship in this era of modern medicine. In the absence of a clear and consistent ethical standard, choices will continue to be made regarding the use of futile therapies, but they will be subject to various abuses. These less-visible approaches may give comfort to those who do not wish to admit or deal with what is already occurring. Yet critics should recognize that, in the final analysis, covert tactics are a more convenient way to dispose of unwanted persons than are openly acknowledged definitions and standards. Explicitly stated criteria and values hold out the promise of evolving toward a more ethical system of health care, one that is in the interest of patients as well as physicians.

CHAPTER EIGHT

The Way It Is Now / The Way It Ought to Be

For Patients

The Way It Is Now

The case of Mary O'Connor, a 77-year-old widow who had a series of progressively debilitating strokes that left her bedridden, with dementia and paralysis, is often cited in ethics and the law as an important case in the evolving debate over the right of family members to refuse unwanted treatment on behalf of patients. It also provided us with one of the earliest insights into the debate over medical futility.

The case entered the courts in 1988, when Mrs. O'Connor's inability to swallow led her doctor at the Westchester County Medical Center to order a nasogastric feeding tube. Her two daughters objected, claiming that such treatment was against their mother's previously and repeatedly expressed wishes that she not be maintained on artificial life support. The New York Court of Appeals, after reviewing the evidence considered by the lower court, concluded that it was not "clear and convincing" that Mrs. O'Connor really knew what she was talking about, despite her background of 20 years working at Jacobi Hospital and confronting severely ill patients on a daily basis; despite her experience of nursing her husband's stepmother, father, and two brothers through long illnesses before they died; and despite her experience with her own hospitalization for congestive heart failure. "There is nothing," the majority concluded, "other than speculation to persuade the factfinder that her expressions were more than an immediate reaction to the unsettling experience of seeing or hearing of another's unnecessarily prolonged death."[1]

Appeals Court Judge Simons wrote a scathing dissenting opinion; it is instructive to view the battle that took place between him and Chief Judge Wachtler, who wrote the majority opinion.

Both judges acknowledged that Mrs. O'Connor was incapable of expressing her treatment wishes because of severe brain damage. Yet, Judge Wachtler concluded that she should receive artificial nutrition through a gastric tube because "death from starvation and especially thirst was a painful way to die and . . . Mrs. O'Connor would, therefore, experience extreme, intense discomfort since she is conscious, alert, capable of feeling pain and sensitive to even mild discomfort."

In his dissent, Judge Simons attacked the very basis for ignoring Mrs. O'Connor's stated wishes on the grounds that they were not "clear and convincing." For who *could* meet such evidentiary standards if a woman with many years of life and considerable experience with illness and health care could not? Mrs. O'Connor had repeatedly expressed her values "in the only terms familiar to her, and she expressed them as clearly as a layperson should be asked to express them, and found 'monstrous' the imposition of artificial means to maintain her under these circumstances."

Simons apparently lacked sufficient medical knowledge to reject Judge Wachtler's most glaring misrepresentation, the use of emotionally stereotyped words such as "thirst" and "starvation," which fails to take into account that dying patients often experience more distress if food and fluids are forced on them—and in any case thirst and starvation can be alleviated by good medical practice and humane care, including pain medications and sedatives.[2] However, he did draw attention to discrepancies between the testimony accepted by the trial court and the distorted descriptions of the patient by Judge Wachtler:

> Preliminarily, it is important to clearly understand the facts of Mary O'Connor's condition. Mrs. O'Connor is a 77-year-old widow who has suffered a series of progressively debilitating strokes that have left her bedridden, substantially

paralyzed and incapable to care for herself. . . . She is neither comatose nor in a vegetative state, but she responds only sporadically to simple questions or commands and then frequently inappropriately. The doctors agree that the neurological damage from the stroke is irreparable and no hope exists for significant improvement in her mental or physical condition. . . . Both daughters testified that since their mother was hospitalized at the medical center, they have visited her daily, sometimes twice a day and, despite their efforts to detect some sign of consciousness, their Mother has never spoken or responded to them in any way even by facial expression or hand movement. . . . This evidence was accepted by the trial court and the Appellate Division and under rules of law too well known to require citation, it binds this court. Nevertheless, the majority [meaning Judge Wachtler's written opinion] characterizes Mrs. O'Connor's condition in quite different terms stating: "She is awake and conscious; she can feel pain, responds to simple commands, can carry on limited conversations, and is not experiencing any pain. She is simply an elderly person who as a result of several strokes suffers certain disabilities, including an inability to feed herself or eat in a normal manner."[3]

Judge Simons pointed out that no reliable witness described Mrs. O'Connor as "conscious" or "alert." He argued that her inability to swallow was

> a substantial loss of a bodily function, analogous to a patient's loss of kidney function requiring dialysis to sustain life or the inability to breathe without the aid of a respirator. Indeed, Mrs. O'Connor cannot even ask to be fed because . . . she could not comprehend that question. . . . While she may not be terminally ill in the sense that death is imminent, she is dying because she has suffered severe injuries to her brain and body, which, if nature takes its course, will result in death. Full medical intervention will not cure or improve her, it will only maintain her in a rudimentary state of existence.[4]

Particularly noteworthy is how Judge Simons ventured beyond mere dissent to invoke a powerful phrase: "a rudimentary state of existence." It seems evident to us that the judge was attempting to grant recognition not only to the values of Mrs. O'Connor as communicated to her daughters, but also to a fundamental value of society, a value that in fact both sides are claiming to represent, one that often is described in abstract terms as "respect for life" or "sanctity of life."[5] This slogan is explicitly or implicitly invoked in virtually every abortion and euthanasia debate. At best it expresses itself in the cautionary query, What safeguards are necessary to prevent the debasement of human life? At worst it shuts off discussion with clamorous references to the Holocaust. Conservatives invoke this principle when they claim that even if a developing fetus is not yet conscious and does not yet have interests of its own, it is nonetheless valuable and merits our dignity and respect. Many conservatives make a parallel claim at the end of life: even if a human being is in permanent vegetative state and ceases forever to be a person with interests and rights, human life itself is precious and worth preserving.

One problem with the sanctity of life principle is that it is often put forward as an ethical absolute that allows for no further ethical dialogue. Properly understood, however, the principle leaves wide open the question of what constitutes showing "proper respect" for human life. In the case of abortion, for example, it is possible to accept the idea that human life is intrinsically valuable while at the same time holding that human life has greater intrinsic value the more fully formed it is, so that a late abortion is more morally troublesome than an early one is. Or someone might endorse the sanctity of life principle, yet interpret it as forbidding bringing into existence a human being who will not be properly nurtured and cared for. The sanctity of life principle is vaguely simplistic and raises more questions than it answers.

But the sanctity of life issue does introduce the inescapable question, Is it possible to honor the wishes of patients like Mrs. O'Connor without plummeting down the slippery slope to a new Nazi era? And one wonders, Did this lurk in the shadow of Judge Wachtler's opinion? And was this the fear that Judge Simons was trying to clear away from the debate?

It is perhaps revealing that Judge Wachtler had to misrepresent the clinical condition of Mrs. O'Connor to claim to protect her sanctity of life *against* any evidence of her wishes. In contrast, Judge Simons accepted both the trial court's description of her clinical condition and the testimony of her wishes as being *most consistent with* protecting her sanctity of life. For, as Judge Simons may have been well aware, Mrs. O'Connor is not alone. Survey after survey has made clear the universality of Mrs. O'Connor's view that it would be "monstrous" to be maintained by medicine in a "rudimentary state of existence." This attitude is shared by every major religious group: 79 percent of Catholics, 70 percent of Jews, and 75 percent of Protestants favor allowing withdrawal of life support from a hopelessly ill or irreversibly unconscious patient. Furthermore, repeated Field Poll surveys have shown that a high percentage of Americans (64% to 75%) support a law that would allow terminally ill patients to obtain life-ending medication.[6] Exceptions in which demands are made to keep an unconscious or barely conscious life going by artificial means are rare. And as we saw in Chapter 4, although such demands may be guided by sincere religious beliefs, it is still hard for families to separate their own emotional and financial considerations from the patient's best interests.

In his dissent, Judge Simons noted regretfully:

> In simpler times, decisions involving life and death were made by the family and its advisers based upon the patient's wishes or what the family thought best as justified by its knowledge of the patient's values and its sense of what the patient's best interests required. In today's world, the sick are removed to hospitals where a broad array of mechanical equipment awaits, capable of prolonging life even though no cure or repair is possible. Necessarily, others must be involved in this decision whether to use it. . . . Few, if any, patients can meet the demanding standard the majority has adopted and the requirements of precision will necessarily be satisfied by pragmatic judicial decisions of what is "best" under the circumstances. . . . The majority, disguising its action as an application of the rule in self-determination, has made its own substituted judgment by improperly finding facts and drawing inferences contrary to the facts found by the courts below. Judges, the persons least qualified by training, experience or affinity to reject the patient's instructions, have overridden Mrs. O'Connor's wishes, negated her long-held values on life and death, and imposed on her and her family their ideas of what her best interest requires.[7]

In the end, society must adjudicate the debate between Judge Wachtler and Judge Simons: What level of human existence is medicine obligated to prolong? For in deciding whether the 77-year-old widow knew what she was talking about, we are deciding what the underlying assumptions of society are. Were her statements so consistent with "long-held values on life and death" by society at large that they could be accepted as clear and convincing evidence? Or were her statements so out of keeping with general societal values that they had to be viewed with extreme suspicion? Here is where the public enters the futility debate.

In previous chapters, we made the case that health providers should not pursue treatments that offer no reasonable chance of benefiting the patient. We argued that physicians are under no obligation to provide such futile treatments, even if demanded. Indeed, we showed that physicians have a positive obligation to avoid harm, to honor a patient's choices among a range of medically beneficial options, and sometimes to say no. Although medicine has great powers, it does not have unlimited powers, and although medicine has great obligations, it does not have unlimited obligations. The duty of the profession is to benefit the patient. Nothing less and nothing more.

In this chapter we turn for the first time to the role that patients and society at large might play in defining the obligations and limits of medicine and the associated standards of medical futility. How can society possibly undertake this task? Is it possible to reach any consensus at all about this contentious issue? The philosopher Daniel Callahan doubts this possibility, stating that there is "no political process to allow physicians and lay people together to develop appropriate standards" for medical futility.[8] Although it is unclear what kind of "political process" Callahan has in mind, he could not realistically expect physicians and society at large to unite spontaneously in supporting a generally accepted definition. Nor, in our opinion, is the well-known process for establishing rationing priorities through town meetings that took place in Oregon readily adaptable to defining futility. Nevertheless, the political process must begin.

Public opinion researcher Daniel Yankelovich points out that in a participatory democracy, it is possible to achieve over time what he calls "public judgment," namely a particular form of public opinion that exhibits "(1) more thoughtfulness, more weighing of alternatives, more genuine engagement with an issue, more taking into account a wide variety of factors than ordinary public opinion as measured in opinion polls, and (2) more emphasis on the normative, valuing, ethical side of questions than on the factual, informational side."[9]

Yankelovich cites several examples of public opinion in which people appear to understand the consequences of their views and have formed relatively stable and consistent judgments. One example is the death penalty. Public polls reveal that since the mid-1960s, more and more people in our country have supported the death penalty, reaching an average of 73 percent favoring the death penalty for murder and other serious crimes in the late 1980s. Interviews with those who support the death penalty reveal that they struggle with the question and are aware of its implications. They recognize, for example, that one implication of instituting a death penalty is that some innocent people will die. Up to now, this awareness has not caused them to change their mind. However, the recent use of new DNA technology to expose erroneous convictions in capital crimes may begin to alter public opinion.

Already, the public discriminates between different circumstances in which the death penalty may be imposed, with fewer people supporting capital punishment for crimes committed by minors or by mentally retarded persons.

Surprisingly, even in the contentious area of abortion, public opinion has demonstrated relative stability over the past 15 years, and the public makes important ethical distinctions. Yankelovich cites a 1989 poll that 49 percent believed that abortion should be legal, 39 percent added critical qualifications, and 9 percent believed that abortion should not be permitted under any circumstances. The stability of public judgment to which Yankelovich refers is in a 2002 Gallup poll looking at attitudes toward abortion in the United States from 1975 through 2002. The poll found that a majority of Americans have almost continually held that abortion should be legal "only under certain circumstances."[10]

Yankelovich likens the gradual emergence of public judgment to a biological process.[11] It begins with dawning awareness of an issue; moves to a sense of urgency and discovery of choices, through wishful thinking; and ends in a more mature stage of taking a stand intellectually and integrating this stand with moral and emotional judgments. When public consensus develops in this manner, and when it reflects "open, inclusive moral discovery and growth,"[12] it solidifies a sense of common purpose and carries moral force in a community.

Yankelovich distinguishes three crucial stages in the evolution of public judgment. The first consists of consciousness raising: the public learns about an issue and becomes aware of its existence and meaning. A second stage in the evolution of public judgment is working through. Working through begins after consciousness is raised, when individuals begin to face the need for change. In the case of medical futility, change must involve altering attitudes and expectations, as well as overt behavior. It requires society to amend widely held expectations about what medicine and science can accomplish. A third stage in the evolution of public judgment is resolution. Resolution is multifaceted and occurs at cognitive, emotional, and moral levels. Cognitive resolution requires people to "clarify fuzzy thinking, reconcile inconsistencies, break down the walls of artificial compartmentalizing that keep them from recognizing related aspects of the same issue, take relevant facts and new realities into account, and grasp the consequences of various choices with which they are presented."[13] Emotional resolution "means that people have to confront their own ambivalent feelings, accommodate themselves to unwelcome realities and overcome their urge to procrastinate and to avoid the issue."[14] Moral resolution involves struggling to do the right thing, even when this requires setting aside one's own needs and desires.

The Way It Ought to Be

We argued in Chapter 3 that physicians, nurses, and other health professionals are responsible for initiating a conversation about medical futility because the professions are given the public trust to define and act in accordance with standards of beneficence. That is, the definition of medical futility must be consistent with the primary goals of medicine and other healing professions, which include benefiting patients. This goal involves limits as well as obligations. Indeed, in Chapter 5 we pointed out why it is important to separate issues of futility from rationing. Yet the fact that health professionals are granted authority to propose standards of medical practice does not imply that society has no role or must passively accept whatever the professions decide.[15]

To the contrary, society functions as the final arbiter of whether the performance of health professionals helps people and benefits society. Where society determines that this has not occurred, society asserts itself and contributes to changing professional behavior by regulating the professions, passing laws to govern professional conduct, or otherwise exerting an influence to alter professional conduct. For example, it is citizens who, in the final analysis, determine whether providing terminally ill, imminently dying patients with a prescription they can use to end their life is consistent with role-related professional standards of care. In the states of Oregon and Washington, citizen initiatives permitting physicians to participate in this practice won approval. In Montana the state supreme court ruled that a prior legislative act regarding withdrawal of treatment for terminally ill patients shielded physicians from prosecution for helping to hasten the death of a consenting, rational, terminal patient.[16]

With respect to medical futility, the process of proposing standards and engaging in conversation and debate is well under way. We have already noted that medical organizations (such as the American Medical Association, the American Heart Association, the Society of Critical Care Medicine, and the American Thoracic Society) and health care facilities now recognize medical futility explicitly and clarify health professionals' responsibilities in this area.

And medical communities and medical societies are also developing consensus standards of care.

In every case, however, the determination that a particular intervention is futile transcends purely empirical medical knowledge. For in every case in which the term *futility* is applied, we either predict that the chance of a significant benefit occurring is so slim that it is futile, or we judge that the qualitative outcome will be so exceedingly poor as to be futile. Yet, as skeptics point out, nothing in physicians' and nurses' medical training prepares them to become experts about ethical matters. Nothing in the study of science teaches a person to know what quality of outcome is worthwhile and what chance of benefit is worth taking. In the domain of ethics, we must assume that health professionals are no better equipped than the next person. If this is correct, why doesn't it follow that health professionals should have no greater authority than patients to assess the ethical aspect of medical futility? Why should not health professionals simply tell their patients what the effects of a particular intervention are likely to be and invite patients to judge for themselves whether those effects count as significant benefits or not? In other words, why shouldn't patients, rather than health professionals, decide the ends of medicine?

We have addressed this question to some extent in Chapter 7, yet at this point we need to explain more fully what role patients should play and why. We begin by noting that medical futility is hardly the only area where medical decisions include ethical components. Value decisions are an ever-present part of the practice of medicine. However, the role of any particular doctor or nurse in setting ethical standards is limited because each is held to standards of the entire medical or nursing profession. The profession as a whole, rather than the individual provider at the bedside, determines the ethical values and purposes of the profession.

Acknowledging that the authority of health professionals to practice medicine and to establish standards of medical care is granted by society suggests that medicine's authority cannot be absolute. Indeed, it always remains contingent on society's continuing to grant its approval. Ultimately, the profession must receive society's sanction to continue to receive the public's trust. If health professionals cease to act for the good of their patients and the society, then their authority will and should be limited. For instance, when the public suspects that physicians are not serving as advocates but are instead promoting their own welfare at the public's expense, medical authority is restricted. When studies showed that physicians who owned their own laboratories and X-ray facilities ordered significantly more tests on their patients than physicians who did not stand to gain from these profit-making facilities, the public was appropriately outraged. Rather than allowing physicians to put their own financial interests ahead of their patients' best interests, the government intervened and regulated physician ownership.

As the health professions reach consensus about the meaning of medical futility, members of society should evaluate this consensus and decide whether or not it is acceptable to them. Physicians and other health professionals can assist the public in reaching cognitive, emotional, and moral resolution by taking the initiative in clearly pointing out alternatives and explaining their consequences. The options we present throughout this book are twofold. One option is for society to require health professionals to offer patients treatments that are unlikely to provide significant benefits. As a consequence of this approach, doctors and nurses would be forced to narrow their understanding of professional responsibility and see the ends of medicine and health care simply as executing patients' wishes, rather than as benefiting patients. Requiring health professionals to provide futile treatment also implies that society must be willing to underwrite the costs of nonbeneficial treatments, spending larger and larger amounts of money on health care.

A second option is for society to assign to health professions the primary responsibility of setting professional standards in this area. This means asking doctors and nurses to renew their commitment to helping patients. Although patients remain free to decide among medically viable options, health professionals would determine what falls inside and outside of professional standards of care. Authorizing health professionals to offer only beneficial treatments, and to limit the use of medically futile options, avoids the high cost associated with applying marginally beneficial technologies. Instead, society's investment in limited health care dollars would be directed to areas where they are of greater benefit.

Getting from Here to There

We close this chapter by issuing a call to action to patients. According to Yankelovich, a successful call to action must include these elements: a vision of what the hoped-for future will look like, specific goals to pursue in reaching that future, strategies for achieving those goals, and techniques for implementing strategies.

A vision. Our vision of health care is patient-centered.[17] It pictures the ends of medicine to include healing the sick and helping and caring for persons. These goals cannot be met by treatments that merely produce physiological effects on an organ system or body part. Instead, medical treatments must provide therapeutic benefits to persons. Keeping a heart beating or lungs breathing does not accomplish medicine's goals when a person will never regain consciousness, or never leave the acute care hospital, or never be free from intense and unremitting pain or misery. A patient-centered approach regards the subject of medical care to be the suffering person, not the biological organism or the failing body part. Specifically, the public must speak out against court decisions that order anencephalic newborns and patients in permanent vegetative state to be kept alive by medical technology.

Specific goals to pursue. The most important goal is for patients and the public to insist that health professionals reaffirm their commitment to benefit patients. As we have noted, evidence suggests that the phenomenon of overtreating patients and acting contrary to conscience is widespread among health professionals, with nearly half (46 percent) of physicians and nurses at five hospitals reporting that they acted against their conscience in providing treatment to critically and terminally ill patients.[18] Patients should no longer tolerate this or accept the high toll it exacts on individuals and families.

Reaffirming a commitment to benefit the patient is an avowal of the oldest ethical traditions of medicine, expressed most eloquently in the Hippocratic writings. Hippocratic medicine teaches that medicine's goal is healing the sick, and this is accomplished through assisting and working with nature. According to Hippocratic ethics, medicine is *techne,* which implies "doing." In doing, one is "bound . . . by the potentialities of the object . . . [and] by those of the *techne* itself."[19]

A second goal that can help to make our vision a reality is for society to insist that health professions conduct and publish empirical research regarding the outcomes of medical treatments on different patient groups, including both positive outcomes (to be achieved) and negative outcomes (to be avoided). Ultimately, knowledge about the outcomes of medical treatments can provide the empirical backing necessary to develop general ethical standards of medical care.

A final goal is for patients to formulate more realistic expectations about what science and medicine can accomplish. Society must face not only the economic limits that scarce health care dollars create but also the technological and human limits inherent in the empirical practice of medicine. Medicine cannot extend human lives indefinitely. Human mortality, which includes pain and suffering, disease and disability, and the certainty of death, cannot simply be conquered by "doing everything."[20]

A strategy to achieve these goals. An effective strategy for achieving the goals stated above requires, first, that the public voice concern about the overuse of medical treatments and insist on accountability from all health professions. Second, public organizations, such as the National Institutes of Health and various Public Health Service agencies that provide important financial backing for clinical research, should be asked to assign a high priority to rigorous, evidence-based outcomes studies. Finally, the public must educate itself about the ethical values that underlie alternative applications of medical technologies. Rather than resorting to an anti-intellectual or antiscience mentality, or engaging in unconstructive technology-bashing, the public should seek to develop a clearer understanding of the ethical values at stake when medical techniques are put to various uses.

Tactics to implement this strategy. The media should be reminded of its professional responsibility to assist with public education and debate. (Just as the medical profession should be taken to task whenever it puts selfish interests ahead of patients' interests, so should the media be challenged whenever it callously sensationalizes events to grab attention and sell products.) Responsible journalism can focus on dramatic cases that crystallize important issues, but it should also include general discussions to identify important misconceptions and solicit input from health care leaders, lawyers, ethicists, economists, and others.

Grassroots civic and educational organizations can also mobilize the public and stimulate a clarification of values through public forums and town meetings that help citizens to wrestle with important social and ethical questions. The *Ethics in America* series broadcast over public television stations is a first-rate example of public education in spirit of "deliberative democracy," which means thoughtful and active citizenship.[21]

In summary, we call on patients to

1. Expect from all health care professionals a renewed commitment to patient-centered medicine—that is, expect a renewed commitment to

heal the sick and help and care for suffering persons. Health professionals should be encouraged to maintain integrity by acting according to a principle of beneficence, or "doing good" for the patient. To
this end, physicians should base decisions on professional standards of
care, rather than on fear of legal liability or because of pressure from
patients and families to "do everything." They should not prolong the
dying process through efforts that merely produce physiological effects
but fail to confer corresponding benefits.

2. Demand that the government, medical schools, hospitals, and other
   institutions direct more attention and funding to improving the
   humane practice of medicine. This emphasis should include both
   empirical research about the outcomes of treatments in different
   patient groups and scholarly ethics research that clarifies the values
   associated with alternative applications of medical technologies.

3. Accept the variety and complexity of the human condition and the
   inevitability of death. This requires acknowledging that there are limits
   to even the most advanced medical and scientific technologies. It also
   entails recognizing that modern medical treatments convey not only
   benefits but also significant psychological, spiritual, and economic
   burdens.

CHAPTER NINE

The Way It Is Now /
The Way It Ought to Be

For Health Professionals

The Way It Is Now

Dora Sauell (not her real name), a widow of some seven years, liked to spend her days bustling from one neighbor to another, keeping up with the latest gossip in the trailer park. One day she awoke with severe chest pain, called 911, and was rushed by ambulance to the emergency department of a nearby hospital, a journey that began a four-month odyssey of complications in the hospital intensive care unit until she died. On admission, a heart attack was diagnosed and treated aggressively with anticoagulants. An attempt was made at coronary angioplasty, in which a catheter is pushed into the coronary artery to open the clot, but this resulted in further damage to the heart muscle, necessitating coronary artery bypass surgery. During her recuperation, Mrs. Sauell developed massive bleeding from a stress ulcer in the stomach. This caused periodic collapses in blood pressure, further damaging her heart and leading also to kidney failure. She then developed a severe respiratory distress syndrome, rendering her unable to breathe and oxygenate her blood without the help of a mechanical ventilator. While in the intensive care unit, she required constant monitoring of blood pressure and heartbeat, correction of electrolytes and supervision of her ventilator, as well as kidney dialysis treatment two to three times a week. Because she continually spiked fevers, the doctors ordered frequent blood cultures. These required repeated punctures of veins that were harder and harder to find. Twice she had a cardiac arrest, and on both occasions her heartbeat was restored by use of a high-voltage cardiac defibrillator. Throughout this time she had fluctuating consciousness, spending most of her time sleeping or grimacing with pain and unable to speak due to the tube in her trachea.

The nurses were in constant turmoil. They regarded their invasive intervention orders as an affront to their compassion for the woman. But whenever they tried to engage the physicians in a discussion about Mrs. Sauell's management, the doctors responded almost angrily to the challenge to their efforts. "Our job is to keep her alive," they would curtly respond.

The several specialists who visited Mrs. Sauell on a daily basis made sure that their treatments were proceeding in the "best" (i.e., most aggressive) fashion. The kidney specialist was satisfied that the schedule of renal dialysis was replacing her lost renal function; the pulmonary specialist was satisfied that the ventilator was maintaining her oxygen level sufficiently high to be compatible with life, and that frequent suctions and occasional bronchoscopies were freeing her of obstructing secretions; the cardiologist concluded that Mrs. Sauell's heart was functioning at maximal capacity even though she was unable to leave the bed. The various specialists therefore believed that their professional duties were being fulfilled. Mrs. Sauell, however, continued to languish in the intensive care unit bed. The problem was that even though each *individual* organ system could be maintained at a marginal level of function by constant intensive treatment, the *combination* of failing organ systems provided overwhelming empirical evidence that the *patient* had only the most negligible chance of ever being rescued from her present disaster.[1]

Finally, the nurses demanded an ethics consultation. After going over the patient and reviewing her medical record, the ethics consulting team reported to the committee their consensus that the patient had no reasonable chance of surviving outside the intensive care unit, that at best she would remain there indefinitely until she experienced some final terminal crisis, most likely a cardiac arrest. The ethics consulting team recommended replacing life-sustaining efforts with comfort care. But then the hospital attorney and the risk manager took over the ethics committee's deliberations. They argued that if the decision to withdraw life-sustaining treatment became known to any of the patient's friends or to the public, the hospital might face embarrassing publicity (or, as they put it, "bad headlines"). Indeed, as long as the patient's insurance was covering the costs of treatment, the balance of benefits versus risks to the hospital clearly lay in continuing the patient's treatment. After considering these points, the ethics committee voted to recommend continuing the present course of treatment.

What we have witnessed in this case is medicine run amok. Body parts are balkanized into subspecialty fiefdoms. The best interests of the hospital prevail over all else. And lost in the swirl is the patient-centered notion of medical treatment. The ethics committee is co-opted by risk managers and hospital attorneys, whose focus in this case was not the good of the patient but the self-interest of the institution. Likewise, the various medical specialists involved in Mrs. Sauell's care took as their focus organ systems, not the patient as a person. "The patient? That's not my department," proclaimed these masters of the kidneys, lungs, heart, and other organs. Wedded to their own technologies, they confused achieving an effect with benefiting a person. "The patient? That's not our client," asserted the hospital attorney and the risk manager. Seeking protective cover for the institution, they persuaded the entire group to continue with futile treatment; in so doing, they became, in the words of ethicist Ruth Macklin, "enemies of patients."[2]

How did this convergence of interests—resulting in Mrs. Sauell's being subjected to months of futile treatments—come about? The physicians, of course, would cite the ideals of their profession as the force motivating their actions. "Our job is to keep her alive," they said.[3] But John B. McKinlay sees a disturbing quality of self-interest in that idealistic proclamation: "With increasing specialization, students and practitioners may be trained to be dependent on certain practices or technologies; hence their continuing livelihood is to some extent contingent on the perpetuation of them. It is understandable, therefore, that some specialties are uncritically committed to particular interventions, and that they vigorously resist attempts to displace and sometimes even to evaluate them."[4]

In other words, not just a narrowly interpreted idealism but an all-too-profitable technological myopia causes specialists to become "uncritically committed to particular interventions," that is, to act like hammers and see every problem as a nail. You can easily imagine that if your specialty is running a mechanical ventilator or a kidney dialysis machine, or performing emergency coronary angioplasty, your first inclination might be to spring to action with your special skill whenever a patient's organ system starts to fail. Only the rare specialist who has the wisdom to raise her sights and view Mrs. Sauell in her entirety will choose a different approach. Rather than forging ahead with useless technologies, such a person will instead withhold aggressive interventions, urging colleagues to do the same, when it is evident that all of their collective efforts will not benefit the patient.

Yet although health professionals in general (and these include hospital attorneys and risk managers) have been entrusted by society to base every professional action on the principle of beneficence, namely, to do only that which is in the best interests of the patient, they sometimes blatantly answer to other needs, as we saw in Mrs. Sauell's case.

In Chapter 6, we witnessed the hypocrisy behind the refusal of the Rush Presbyterian St. Luke's Medical Center to withdraw the life-sustaining ventilator from the permanently unconscious baby, Sammy Linares. While stoutly maintaining that they could not participate in the heinous act of killing the baby, the hospital authorities said they would find no difficulty in removing the ventilator if Mr. Linares, the father, obtained a court order. In a similar example of sanctimony, Grace Plaza nursing home wrote in a letter to the husband of Jean Elbaum, dunning him for unwanted services, that they could not withdraw a life-sustaining feeding tube from his wife, who had severe dementia, because of "an overriding interest in continuing life support, irrespective of the patient's wishes." Yet in the very same letter the director warned, "You may be aware that New York State regulation sanctions the discharge of a patient for non-payment."[5] In other words, their "overriding" dedication to the preservation of life would not be a barrier to kicking out a woman in financial arrears and letting her die somewhere else!

Even if we accept the idealistic claims of health providers, it is becoming a matter of increasing embarrassment that physicians are failing to support all their therapeutic claims, namely, failing to justify their treatments by empirical evidence demonstrating patient benefit. As the physician and health policy expert David Eddy points out: "We are still relying on personal observations and uncontrolled clinical series, mixed together with heavy doses of clinical judgment, to learn the outcomes of our practices. These methods are simply not up to the task of evaluating modern medical practices." In fact, after surveying the medical literature, the Congressional Office of Technology Assessment concluded that only 10 to 20 percent of medical treatments in current use are supported by randomized trials. As a result, says Eddy, "we are uncertain about outcomes, there are wide variations in practice patterns, a large proportion of practices appear to be inappropriate, the evidence for most procedures is poor, and there are uncontrollable increases in costs."[6]

In a scathing commentary entitled "Technology Follies," the physician David Grimes takes his colleagues to task for not "requiring rigorous evidence of efficacy or validity before adoption and dissemination of new technologies." And although we have concentrated on life-saving technologies, we emphasize that the ethical standard of patient benefit applies to all medical treatments. Reviewing a kaleidoscope of prevalent practices—postcoital sperm survival tests of infertility; electronic fetal monitoring; episiotomy in childbirth; chemotherapeutic, immunologic, and physical methods to purge tumor cells before bone marrow transplantation; radial keratotomy to correct refractive errors of the eye—of all these and other new or venerable practices, Dr. Grimes asks rhetorically: "What procedures or practices are we involved in now which will rank with bloodletting as a folly of our time?" As Dr. Grimes observes, "'new' is not synonymous with 'improved.' This confusion, coupled with poor scientific standards, has squandered resources, wasted effort, and in some cases, harmed or killed our patients."[7]

Physician Stephen Schoenbaum points out that between 1980 and 1990, the procedures performed on the patient in our example (Mrs. Sauell) increased dramatically overall: coronary bypass surgery more than doubled, and percutaneous transluminal coronary angioplasty increased more than ninefold. "One might expect that this phenomenon would be accompanied by a marked improvement in outcome for the American population," Schoenbaum says. Yet he notes that groups who were less likely to undergo these procedures, such as women and blacks, had at least as good a chance, or a better chance, of survival.[8]

But desperate patients and their advocates cry, How will medicine ever discover new treatments and achieve new breakthroughs if it doesn't keep applying new interventions? Here we have to acknowledge that the medical profession, government agencies like the Food and Drug Administration, and society at large, particularly activists fighting particular diseases, often fail to draw an important distinction between treatments that empirically have already been shown to fail and therefore should be considered futile, and treatments for which there is promising but as yet insufficient supportive evidence and therefore can be regarded as experimental.

With respect to unproven but plausible treatments, physician-ethicist Steven Miles raises an appropriate caution:

> Our society believes that technical progress will solve tragic problems. Entrepreneurs and researchers implicitly or explicitly promise such relief. Many desperately ill persons choose to participate in creating medical progress or reaping its first, most uncertain, benefits. The recent controversy over government procedures for releasing unproven AIDS treatments for clinical use illustrates the power of these values. Permitting private purchase of nonvalidated therapies (e.g. for-profit, noninsured immunotherapy for cancer) both undercuts the definition of futility and poses a complex problem for fair access for progress itself.[9]

We would add that the confusion may stem from society's optimistic but erroneous belief that any new treatment that comes along is more likely to succeed than to fail. As a result, there is always enthusiasm and pressure to try a new drug or a gleaming new machine just seen in a two-minute spot on the nightly news. But this assumption that something new is likely to succeed is undermined by the more sobering empirical data. To cite one important example, the Pharmaceutical Manufacturers Association reports that for every 5,000 chemically synthesized substances, only 250 reach the stage of animal testing, 5 are studied in humans, and only 1 ends up being approved by the Food and Drug Administration.[10] In short, at every step of development most new drugs are cast aside. Moreover, FDA approval by no means is the end of the story. From 1975 to 1999, even after being approved by the FDA, more than 10 percent of drugs were forced to display a hitherto unanticipated new black box warning or were withdrawn because of serious adverse drug events. During the following period of 1998-2005, the rate of reported deaths and serious injuries increased more than twofold.[11]

Physician and researcher Thomas Chalmers estimates that, with the rare exception of the discoveries of penicillin for pneumonia, vitamin B_{12} for pernicious anemia, insulin for diabetic acidosis, and perhaps one or two other situations in the whole history of medicine, fewer than one out of a thousand new treatments introduced every year turns out to be unequivocally successful. Most are of limited, dubious, or negligible benefit or, indeed, may be harmful.[12]

Thus, we emphasize that although patients certainly are entitled to ask their doctors for the opportunity to participate in an ongoing randomized clinical trial of an experimental drug or procedure that is promising, they do not have a right to demand as *therapy* that for which there is no demonstrated benefit or that for which there is overwhelming empirical evidence that it will not succeed. (We distinguish between the word *treatment,* whose root meaning is to "handle" or "deal with," and *therapy,* whose root meaning is to "cure.") Once again, medications and procedures with no demonstrated benefits should be regarded as experimental until their benefits or their futility are shown through objective, prospective, randomized clinical trials. Patients receiving unproven treatments outside a formal clinical trial are participating in misguided experiments and should be so advised by physicians who offer such treatments; they will not be protected by institutional human subject review boards that monitor all bona fide research on patients.

The way it is now, this does not always happen. For, as Dr. Chalmers reports:

> Unfortunately, when a physician decides he has an exciting new therapy, he usually feels he cannot start a control trial immediately because he is not sure of the dose and the patient to select; so he does a pilot study of consecutive patients. That prevents him from ever doing a randomized controlled trial for one of three reasons: He is so impressed with the efficacy of the drug in the uncontrolled trial that he cannot do a study for ethical reasons, and he publishes his "excellent results" in a preliminary paper. He concluded that a control trial should be done but he does not do it because he is convinced that the drug works. It is often ten years before other clinical investigators, stimulated by a lack of success and less well patients, report equally uncontrolled negative series or finally do a controlled trial. A second possibility is that the originator of the therapy cannot do a control trial because the treatment seems so ineffective that he cannot subject more people to it; yet it is entirely possible that it is the selection of patients who receive the treatment rather than the treatment itself that is at fault. This is especially true in the case of drastic "last resort" therapies. . . . At any rate, the therapy appears so unfavorable that a controlled trial would be unethical. The third possibility is that the therapy appears to be similar to other therapies, and the investigator has no incentive to spend his time doing a control trial to prove that a suggestive therapy is no different from the standard. . . . the only way to avoid this trap is to randomize the first patients.[13]

As we previously noted, Mildred Solomon and colleagues reported the astonishing fact that a majority of doctors had participated in treatments which they regarded as inappropriate for terminally ill patients but which they nevertheless continued to force on their patients in spite of pangs of conscience.[14] It is distressing to have observed politicians during the debate over the Obama administration's health care reform proposals distort and smear evidence-based medicine, referring to effectiveness research as "pulling the plug on granny."

Because of their location in the hierarchy of power, nurses suffer particularly from this cognitive and moral dissonance. This dissonance, described as "moral distress," is the emotional suffering one undergoes when forced to act in a way that one recognizes to be wrong. The nurses caring for Mrs. Sauell were particularly vulnerable. Every day they were at the patient's bedside, witnesses to her misery, nausea, or incontinence; yet, despite their misgivings about treatments, they felt responsible for abiding by orders to attend to the patient's intravenous and nasogastric tubes and mechanical ventilators, and to assist with cardiac resuscitation. Throughout the process of caring for Mrs. Sauell, nurses may have felt powerless to change the patient's circumstances because the physicians had ordered them to follow certain procedures and because the hospital authorities had overruled their concerns.

Nurse and researcher Judith M. Wilkinson surveyed and interviewed some two dozen hospital nurses and discovered that almost all of them had experienced this kind of moral distress at least once a week. These experiences produced anger, frustration, and guilt; some nurses believed that the quality of the care they delivered was compromised. Most cases associated with moral distress for nurses involved activities that caused pain and suffering to patients or required treating patients in what was perceived as a dehumanizing way. To review their comments on the patients they cared for is in itself distressing. For example:

> The man was a century old. He would probably have gone in peace and would not have had to spend his last days this way—he has decubitus, an open sore. He has been on the ventilator, comatose, in this state forever.

> I remember crying as we cleaned her up. There was a lot of blood. They had tried to start IVs and stuff. She was oozing blood; she had started vomiting as she stopped breathing. Dark fluid . . . was coming out of her mouth. Her abdomen was distended and tight—probably full of blood. She looked bad. I just felt she should have been able to die with some kind of dignity.[15]

How do physicians get lured into prescribing treatments that offer no benefit to their patients and yet persist in pursuing these measures? Again, we go to Dr. Chalmers. He points out that as far back as 1969, physicians had information warning them that oral drugs that lowered blood glucose were more likely than either an inactive placebo or insulin to cause the death of their diabetic patients. Although the prevailing idea at the time was that lowering blood glucose would save lives by reducing the rate of cardiovascular disease in patients with diabetes, a prospective clinical study showed that, quite the contrary, the drugs seemed to increase the risk of death. The results were met with great controversy, and it was generally agreed that further studies were necessary. But none were undertaken. "Meanwhile," writes Dr. Chalmers, "as a result of the 'ethical practice' of medicine, gross sales of oral agents have steadily climbed. The only conclusion one can draw is that we should have had multiple studies started simultaneously when the drugs were first introduced, so we could answer the therapeutic questions before the ethical problems became insurmountable."[16]

This is yet another example of conflating the ideas of "effect" and "benefit," a problem that is perhaps an expected outcome of medical training. Physicians' training tends to focus on effects achieved on body parts (such as hearts, lungs, and blood glucose) as distinct from benefits experienced by the patient as a person. Because of early studies, diabetes specialists assumed that strict control of blood glucose would improve a patient's health and prolong life by preventing complications such as cardiovascular disease, blindness, and kidney failure. They assumed that producing a physiological effect (lowering blood glucose) was equivalent to achieving a benefit for the patient (preventing complications and prolonging life). In fact, years after Dr. Chalmers' warning, studies confirm that strict control of blood glucose fails to reduce adverse cardiovascular outcomes and either increases or has no effect on mortality; moreover, it increases the risk for severe hypoglycemia in type 2 diabetes.[17]

Another example of effect-benefit confusion that proved harmful, even fatal, occurred when physicians imprudently began prescribing erythropoietin, a red cell growth factor, based on the results of a few small, uncontrolled studies that showed that the medication raised blood levels to a "normal" range in anemic patients with cancer and chronic kidney disease. Once again, this physiological effect on the blood was assumed to be beneficial. Unfortunately, when carefully designed clinical trials were carried out comparing the intervention to a placebo control, the treatment resulted in significantly more harm to patients, including stroke, heart attack, hospitalization, and death.[18]

The Way It Ought to Be

There are signs that critics within medicine are losing patience with the current state of their profession and are raising serious doubts that physicians have lived up to their ethical responsibilities. Dr. Stephen Schoenbaum, for example, states:

> It should be disturbing to us as a profession that we have so few outcomes data and use so few in our practices. . . . And although we talk about *primum non nocere* [first to do no harm] we clearly have a bias toward action. It is hard to escape the fact that we can rejoice with our patients and their families when they have good outcomes, empathize with them when they have poor outcomes, get personal gratification from the interaction and our work in both instances, and not trouble them or ourselves with hard data. In short, we learn to enjoy playing the game of medical care without hard evidence and the outcome—often unknown in statistical terms—is of secondary importance to the process.[19]

Like his colleague, Dr. McKinlay, Schoenbaum then issues a more devastating indictment:

> Major industries have grown up to support our practices. The industry supporting angiography—PTCA [percutaneous transluminal coronary angioplasty] and bypass surgery—ranges from medical equipment companies to the educational apparatus that trains all the levels of staff engaged in the decision-making and execution of these procedures to the hospitals and surgicenters whose bottom lines depend on this production. They are formidable forces with which to contend.[20]

The evolution of clinical practice guidelines is a visible manifestation of the shift away from relying exclusively on the "bias toward action" every time a patient seeks medical help and toward examining more forthrightly whether or not the medical intervention will provide a benefit. At best, these guidelines are the product of expert panels that review the accumulated evidence associated with a particular intervention and provide a consensus statement and set of recommended practices along with a critical appraisal of the evidence in support of the panel's recommendations. At worst, they are biased pep talks by advocates from industry, medical specialties, or disease affinity groups that place their own interests and ideology over empirical data—as recently seen in the screening mammogram controversy.[21]

The best guidelines are based on the notion of technology assessment, which seeks to improve the care of individual patients by gathering and analyzing information from studies carried out on large groups of patients. Even so, critics have faulted many of these studies for reflecting the scientific perspective of statisticians rather than the perspectives of patients. For example, a popular booklet put out by the American Heart Association reported the death rate of patients with coronary heart disease, but nowhere mentioned what George Diamond and Timothy Denton call "the plight of the survivors—their level of disability and quality of life." Diamond and Denton continue: "Similarly, much technology assessment is based on physician-oriented 'objective' outcomes such as physical signs and test responses, rather than patient-oriented 'subjective' outcomes such as quality of life and well-being. Objective outcomes are certainly easier for investigators to measure, but subjective outcomes are arguably more relevant to individual patients."[22]

According to the American College of Physicians, "When done well—as some indisputably are—guidelines seem to represent the best possible way to collect, make sense of and then summarize for otherwise overwhelmed doctors the abundance of current research and opinion on medical procedures and outcomes."[23] The college warned, however, that nearly every group with a stake in health care is busily writing guidelines, including physician specialty societies, insurance companies, utilization reviewers, patient advocacy groups, and managed care organizations. Although the putative purpose of such guidelines is to provide the best and most appropriate patient care, some groups may be more interested in justifying procedures, reimbursements, or cost-cutting measures or promoting business or other private interests. Therefore, it is essential that physicians demand that any expert panels provide background information to their recommendations, including whether or not those recommendations are based on well-controlled, randomized studies, or on less rigorous evidence. Equally important, physicians should require that outcome measures take benefiting the patient as a focus and goal, rather than producing effects on body parts.

Dr. Bruce G. Charlton relates this demand for evidence-based medicine to a growing public health orientation within bioethics. He points out that although bioethics was traditionally concerned with the moral code regulating the doctor-patient relationship, public health views this relationship within the context of the community as a whole and in light of scientific measures that enhance society's health. According to Charlton, "In public health, it is generally untrue to say that something *must* be done, because if there is no good scientific evidence of benefit, then it is better that *nothing* be done. Scientific evidence for a treatment's effectiveness should be established *before* it is introduced into the medical setting on a large scale" (italics in original).[24] The same logic applies on a small scale: when there is no scientific evidence that *something* benefits an individual patient, it is better that *nothing* be done to that patient.

It should not come as a surprise that there are those in medicine and other health care professions who are nervous about appearing in public without the clothes of the emperor. Are we really capable of looking at ourselves critically? Clearly, some of us are, for we recognize that if the public draws attention to our raiment—some sequins, some patches—before we do, embarrassment will be the least of our worries. Society rightly reacts with outrage when it senses a conspiracy to hide the truth. And although such skepticism is generally salutary, it sometimes provokes irrational reactions. In the case of medicine, these suspicions have contributed to literally thousands of patients' undergoing unnecessary suffering and premature death because they did not trust the medical profession or its warnings about many ruthlessly promoted quack cancer cures.

There can be little doubt that modern medicine offers powerful therapies to the sick. At the same time, much of what physicians do emerges from habit, conventional wisdom, and authority, and lacks that most valuable quality—supportive empirical evidence. Fortunately, medicine today is undergoing a major change, recognizing the need "to make an orderly transition to a world based on evidence, carefully designed processes of care, and truly informed consent."[25]

There are indications also that physicians are reexamining their relationships with patients and their understandings of medicine's goals. Sometimes these inquiries lead to startling results. Along with other researchers, we discovered that physicians do a poor job predicting what their patients would want in terms of various life-sustaining treatments.[26] The physicians are not alone; husbands and wives also are not very good at predicting what their spouses would want.[27] But even more disquieting, we discovered that physicians tend to project their own values on their patients.[28] Another group of physicians, led by Dr. John Wennberg, showed that patients facing prostatectomy (surgical removal of the prostate in an effort to cure cancer or partial removal to alleviate symptoms of enlargement) who were exposed to an interactive videotape answering questions and offering patients' testimonials agreed to the surgery much less often than those patients who had only been exposed to the advice of their surgeon.[29]

Using this educational methodology, Dr. Wennberg and colleagues went to great efforts to obtain *informed* consent from patients. But what about patients who are not so well informed, indeed who are influenced by the self-serving, promotional efforts of physicians and health care industry leaders who advertise their wares with enthusiasm rather than with rigorous supporting clinical data—as is happening with robot-assisted prostate surgery? This rapidly growing technology requires the hospital to invest in a $1.2 million machine and a $140,000 annual service contract (a strong incentive to garner patient fees) without clear evidence that it provides superior outcomes to patients with cancer. Although robotically assisted surgical patients possibly have shorter hospital stays and complications (a boon to for-profit hospitals receiving Medicare case–based single payments), they are likely to experience more impotence and incontinence (not such a boon for patients who might regard these outcomes as more important). Nevertheless, "doctors and medical centers advertise it, and patients demand it," reported the Harvard physician Michael J. Barry, creating a "folie à deux."[30] Thus, it is clear that physicians have a responsibility to provide clear, objective information—including the fact of uncertainty—to their patients. Failing to do this, in our opinion, is unconscionable. In addition to providing this information, physicians should be sensitive not only to the values patients hold, especially where benefits are problematic, but also to the impact their own personal and professional values have on what passes for their patients' "voluntary" choices.

What will the public's reaction be to this demythologizing of medicine? We recognize that some segments of the public may stubbornly refuse to accept any limits on their demands for treatments, no matter how useless those treatments might be.[31] Yet more care is not always better care. Sometimes, in fact, it's worse.[32] As we noted above, the debate over screening mammography for breast cancer in women under the age of 50 is a good example. Although 30 years of studies have found no evidence that screening younger women without risk factors saves lives, some advocates demand that the X-ray test be included in health care plan benefits for younger women anyway. The declarations of Amy Langer, executive director of the National Alliance of Breast Cancer Organizations, exemplifies how easily the issue can be politically manipulated from one of medical value to one of symbolic significance. "What you have now," she argues, "is a very powerful group of women who are extremely angry and frustrated that very little is known about breast cancer." Ignoring the data in her misguided anger, she continues: "Women will not stand for the government or others to try to take away the only tool we have that is a proven intervention. Maybe it's not good enough, but it's the best we have."[33] While well intentioned, this approach is misguided. The use of mammography in younger women without risk factors may even cause more harm than good, because the vast majority of "positive" findings are false, leading to unnecessary anxiety while the women undergo additional procedures including breast biopsies. More disturbingly, early reports raise the concern that exposure to radiation from annual mammograms on young women *without* risk factors may even *increase* the risk of cancer.[34]

Generally speaking, the process of open and honest scrutiny can unleash unsophisticated outcries, which, abetted by special interests and clumsy political action, may result in more harm than good to society. But our response is, first, to underscore society's right to be informed about all aspects of medical care and, second, to be optimistic about the marketplace of ideas and hopeful that public discussion will in the long run lead an educated society to make thoughtful and worthy choices.

Already, law professor Alan Meisel has seen a public consensus developing in support of medical approaches that replace aggressive, pointless treatments with an acceptance of limits and an emphasis on compassion. He points out that "the consensus about the circumstances under which it is legitimate to forgo life-sustaining treatment has become as widely accepted as it is in no small part because it has found a receptive audience among judges, legislators, and the public at large whose views lawmakers often reflect."[35]

Indeed, evidence of this can be seen in the popular press. For example, the *New York Times* reported approvingly:

> Already, medical researchers are trying to reduce ineffective or harmful procedures by developing guidelines on, for example, which patients will benefit from operations like coronary bypass. Insurers, through "managed care," have also tried to weed out procedures and hospital days that are not medically necessary.
>
> Pruning out inappropriate care is only sensible—but it is not rationing. Refusing to pay for something, not because it is ineffective but because its costs greatly outweigh potential benefits, would be the great departure.[36]

Not every expert agrees that rationing is ethically necessary or justified, even if the country seeks to curb spending. After studying the results of many procedures—including coronary bypass, angioplasty, hysterectomy, and gall bladder operations—Dr. Robert Brook and his colleagues at the Rand Corporation concluded that one-quarter to one-third of all medical care in the country is either inappropriate or carries risks that equal potential benefits. "We have to get rid of all that before we talk about rationing," Dr. Brook said.[37]

Or, as Jane E. Brody, a medical writer for the *New York Times*, said, "Families as well as patients are often furious and frustrated with what they consider a lack of compassion in medicine's insistence upon prolonging a life that no longer seems worth living."[38]

It seems clear to us, therefore, that health professionals must take the lead in establishing ethical limits to their obligation to attempt treatments that empirical evidence shows are destined to be futile. Dr. David Mirvis, exhorting his medical colleagues to speak "with one voice," points out that medicine is based on a highly specialized body of knowledge that is not easily accessible to the public. Mirvis notes that "even though the public does not fully understand what the profession does," society trusts physicians to act in the public's best interest; society looks to the institutions of medicine for the establishment of "codes of ethics, expectations of physicians' practice standards, and fundamental mechanisms for peer review, as well as basic standards of medical education." Physicians, he admonishes, "can give the patients only that which they have under their control."[39]

Where Do We Go from Here?

At the outset of this book we noted that although the term *futility* is actively used in medical discourse, some critics object to the concept, calling it "elusive," "unsettling," "dangerous," and devoid of a "clear sense of public values."[40] If such objections prevail, they will effectively undermine assertions made over many years by a wide variety of authorities that physicians are not obligated to provide futile treatment.[41] Must medical futility be construed only as an ambiguous concept, cited in the abstract, or can it be defined with sufficient specificity to be useful in clinical practice?

As we have noted, much of the resistance to the notion of futility derives from the fear that it will serve as a masquerade for less defensible motivations. For example, will its acceptance revive the discarded abuses of medical paternalism? Will it reverse recent advances in patient autonomy and shared decision-making? Will the power to declare treatment futile provide a convenient excuse for physicians to neglect patients they deem unworthy? Will it entice nervous health care providers to avoid patients with life-threatening contagious illness? Will futility serve as a devious rationale for reducing medical costs?

We acknowledge these potential corruptions of the concept, yet maintain that they are more likely to occur if professional groups and health care institutions *fail* to establish clear guidelines. Only by developing a rigorous definition of futility can we protect patients and families from abuse (which includes both refusing to offer beneficial treatment and refusing to withdraw futile interventions). It is particularly important, for example, to distinguish futility (implying no apparent therapeutic benefit) from rationing (acknowledging therapeutic benefit but raising questions about availability and costworthiness).[42] In our experience, rationing is the notion most often confused with futility. For just as physicians find it painful to admit to a patient or family that they have run out of beneficial treatments, so too they find it difficult to upset egalitarian ideals by selectively apportioning such treatments.

Not too long ago, a period of uncertainty preceded the establishment of a uniform definition of death based on the so-called whole brain standard. After considerable public debate and expert debate and testimony within the medical, philosophical, and legal communities, most states adopted the Uniform Brain Death Act.[43] Although it is unlikely that the definition of futility will ever be enshrined at the statutory level (nor should it, because it inherently depends on a complex variety of clinical circumstances and treatments), we propose that professional groups define the therapeutic futility of specific medical interventions in conjunction with evolving "standards of care" for those interventions.

Just as we use empirical studies to gather data about treatments that provide significant clinical benefits, we should also be paying attention to treatments that do not provide such benefits.[44] The development of clinical predictive models in intensive care units for critically ill children and adults is an important recent medical advance that offers physicians the opportunity to forecast and distinguish with increasing accuracy survivors and nonsurvivors. Examples of such models employing various clinical and laboratory measures are APACHE (Acute Physiology, Age, Chronic Health Evaluation), SOFA (Sequential Organ Failure Assessment), and PRISM (Pediatric Risk of Mortality).[45]

These were developed on the basis of experience with thousands of patients and were validated in many different ICUs in at least six different countries. More recently, investigators took into account the dynamic nature of disease and added a time dimension to the scoring system to enhance the accuracy of prediction.

Skeptics have argued that the use of scoring systems for seriously ill patients, though offering overall probabilities, are nonetheless limited in their power to predict futility in a particular patient. However, physicians are not limited to numerical scores in predicting futility. Many conditions cannot be overcome, and physicians can often reasonably conclude at some clinical stage that there is no realistic chance the patient will benefit from aggressive treatment. Although scoring systems cannot predict a treatment outcome with absolute certainty, they provide valuable information about its likelihood. Such information has already provided the empirical basis for establishing standards of care, which refer not only to the employment of useful treatments but also to the withholding of useless ones.[46]

With the availability of standards of care to serve as clinical practice guidelines for physicians and as professional standards for the courts, physicians who decline to use futile treatments, even when demanded by patients and families, will be able to make these decisions with legal, ethical, and community support.

Getting from Here to There

So far we have emphasized that a wide gulf exists between the way things are and the way things ought to be. We now turn to the practical problem of getting from here to there. Throughout this book, we emphasize that changing the practice of medicine so that futile treatments are no longer applied requires the medical profession to achieve consensus about the definition of medical futility. We now wish to add the important point that, in the last analysis, society at large must understand and approve of any definition of futility and accept or reject the ethical implications proposed in this book.

The distinction we draw between effects and benefits requires for its application not only empirical data, but also ethical assessments of when effects represent benefits or harms to patients. We can look to the empirical practice of medicine to provide information about the outcomes of various interventions in different populations. Initially, medicine and other health care professions bear the responsibility of formulating professional standards in this area.[47] These professions are accountable to the public which they serve, of course, and the public must ultimately decide whether or not it agrees that particular outcomes provide an ethically acceptable likelihood or quality of benefit to persons or are futile.

In this regard, it is instructive to review the debate that ensued when we called on the American Heart Association (AHA) to modify the professional standards for emergency medical service units attempting CPR and other life-prolonging treatments outside the hospital setting.[48] Under the then-existing AHA standards, paramedics responding to an emergency call were obligated to attempt CPR—even when it was clearly futile—unless the victim showed grossly obvious signs of death, such as decapitation, rigor mortis, or the changes of tissue decomposition and discoloration. We pointed out that in other areas of medicine, decisions are made to withhold a futile treatment without requiring that the patient be dead. Why cannot attempted CPR decisions similarly be made in accordance with a patient-centered notion of medical futility—that is, in accordance with whether or not under the circumstances attempted CPR is likely to restore the patient, at the very least, to conscious awareness?

Although acknowledging that "physicians should not be obligated to provide futile therapy when asked to do so by patients or surrogates," the AHA rejected what it called a "less strict and less objective" and "looser meaning of futility." The examples it gave to counter the "less strict and less objective" application of medical futility are sadly revealing of how medicine has lost its way. CPR, stated the AHA, should always be attempted in a young patient in a permanent vegetative state because even though it will not restore consciousness, it may restore circulation and therefore permit long-term survival. And, stated the AHA, CPR should never be withheld unless "no survivors have been reported under given circumstances in well-designed studies."[49] Fortunately, as we noted previously, a more reasonable guideline has been recently proposed that may supersede the earlier AHA guideline.[50]

It should be clear from these examples that terms like *strict* and *loose* are imprecise and misleading. The debate over whether CPR should be attempted to preserve a permanently unconscious body is not a matter of strict or loose criteria, but of whether such an outcome is an appropriate goal of medicine. One can set strict criteria that focus on patient-centered benefits and exclude the goal of preserving unconscious biological existence. Similarly, the requirement that paramedics or physicians attempt CPR unless "no survivors" were reported in "well-designed" studies includes both an absurdity and a hidden value statement. As we have already pointed out in Chapter 1, one can never be absolutely certain under any circumstances that there will be zero survivors. Furthermore, what value assumptions are hidden in the term "well-designed" study? Does it mean one that draws conclusions after a hundred cases, a thousand cases, a million cases? At some point, common sense (we hope) will step in and say, "Enough's enough!" But when this happens, it will not be in accordance with some objective, "strict" criteria, but rather when the medical profession, supported by society, agrees that a treatment was tried enough times, and shown not to achieve the intended benefit to the patient.

Interestingly, lawyers (more than physicians) are sometimes in the vanguard of seeking to prevent the legal chaos of ad hoc and patchwork court decisions by establishing standards of care regarding medical futility.[51] Because courts look to statements by professional groups and institutions for definitions of standards of practice and of the legal duties to which members of the medical professions must comply, publicly stated institutional policies regarding medical futility will be important to protect and reassure physicians and those who seek to override demands for futile treatment. Otherwise, says law professor Marshall B. Kapp, "the legal system will continue to blunder along with physicians dragged in tow."[52]

In a section of a law review article entitled "Why Hospitals Should Adopt a Policy on Futility," Professor Lance Stell states:

> Hospitals should consider adopting clear, reasonable institutional standards for withholding or withdrawing futile treatments that would serve as a local standard of care. These standards should require prompt, clear communication with the patient or his representative regarding withholding or withdrawing interventions on grounds of futility. Not to do this invites suspicion and cynicism and erodes medical integrity. In the absence of a standard, physicians who feel compelled to comply with medically unjustified demands for full measures may practice strategic concealment of their decisions or deliver half-measures in selected cases.[53]

Because all of us, both health professionals and laypeople, may at some time be patients who are subject to the definition and ethical principles that govern medical futility, we all have an essential stake in developing a definition and associated ethical principles about futility. For these reasons, health care professionals are responsible to educate patients and the public at large about the meaning and ethical implications of medical futility.

In particular, society and the medical profession should not be lured into the position that "it's only a matter of money," with the implication that no standards or limits should be set, but rather should affirm that doctors and those in the other healing professions should not be expected to do anything, no matter how extreme and absurd, as long as someone is willing to pay for it. Apparently, as we pointed out in Chapter 5, the *New York Times* viewed the futility debate in this simplistic way when it headlined the story about a hospital's efforts to discontinue what it regarded as inappropriate life-prolonging treatment of an anencephalic infant (born with most of its brain missing): "Court Order to Treat Baby Prompts a Debate on Ethics: At What Point Does Treatment Cease to Be Worth the Expense?" Is this what the health care profession wants: to uphold, like the oldest profession, no standards other than those of the marketplace?

In proposing the quantitative component of futility, we tried to overcome the problem of uncertainty in medicine by asking whether or not physicians would agree with the commonsense notion that if a treatment has not benefited the patient in the last 100 cases, it would be reasonable to conclude that it is futile (upper limit of 95% confidence interval = 3%).[54] Because this standard comports with what has become the traditionally conservative level of medical inference of statistical significance, expressed as $p < 0.01$, it is probably not surprising that other physicians independently arrived at a similar quantitative threshold when invoking futility on an empirical basis.[55]

We acknowledge that the actual application of the quantitative component of futility will probably vary in different communities and hospitals because the likelihood of a patient with complex and serious illness surviving to hospital discharge following attempted CPR will not necessarily be the same in a small rural hospital as it is in a major urban teaching center. Nor will the combinations of patient characteristics associated with survival following attempted CPR (e.g., diseases, age, gender) be the same in all hospitals.[56] This does not mean, however, that the definition of futility itself varies. Nor does it mean that medical futility should be defined so loosely as to escape professional standards.

Although we do not anticipate a "national futility policy" consisting of a single, universal practice guideline, we are encouraged to see that the medical profession throughout the country is addressing the issues of medical futility's meaning and ethical implications and is establishing consensus standards of care. For example, at the community level, representatives from 11 San Diego area hospitals comprising the San Diego Bioethics Commission—including a major university hospital, a Veterans Administration hospital, several large health maintenance organizations, a military hospital, and a Catholic hospital—came together and after a year of discussions adopted a model benefit–based futility policy. At the state level, the California Medical Association urged adoption and recommendation to the American Medical Association of a clearly defined "nonbeneficial treatment" policy in support of the AMA Code of Medical Ethics of 1996, which declares, "All health care institutions, whether large or small, should adopt a policy on medical futility." Most recently, in 2009, the AMA took a significant step further when they adopted Resolution 003, "Limiting Futile Care at End of Life": "RESOLVED, That our American Medical Association seek legislation by the United States Congress that will allow the creation of a methodology directed by physicians (MDs/DOs) that permits physicians (MDs/DOs) to either not engage in or to suspend futile care at the end of life; and that those physicians (MDs/DOs) be given immunity from liability when such decisions are made in good faith and within the standard of care with clear and convincing legal and ethics standards."[57]

And at the federal level, the Uniform Health-Care Decisions Act lends further support: "A health care provider or institution may decline to comply with an individual instruction or health care decision that requires medically ineffective health care or health care contrary to generally accepted health care standards applicable to the provider or the health care institution."[58] To intercept any doubt, the act further explains that " 'medically ineffective health care' as used in this section, means treatment which would not offer the patient any significant benefit."[59]

These professional bodies agree that medical futility refers to treatments that have no reasonable chance of benefiting the patient. As we have suggested, although variables such as age, gender, and diseases may not be reliable predictors in all hospitals, they most likely will be reliable across the majority of institutions. Therefore, specific protocols for withholding and withdrawing CPR could be tailored to individual institutions, as long as professional standards of care are met.

Both quantitative and qualitative components of medical futility highlight the distinction between a treatment effect, which merely alters some part of the patient's body, and a treatment benefit, which can be appreciated by the patient and enables the patient to escape total dependence on the acute care hospital. With respect to qualitative futility, a treatment that cannot provide a minimum level of benefit should be regarded as futile. Neither qualitatively futile nor quantitatively futile treatments are owed to the patient as a matter of moral duty. To the contrary, the physician has a positive duty to cease or withhold futile interventions.

Although we are heartened to see this growing consensus, we acknowledge that there is as yet no universal agreement on a single definition of medical futility. We have observed, however, that this lack of unanimity has not kept the term from being invoked by health providers to justify decisions concerning treatment or nontreatment. In consultations and conferences we occasionally hear futility cited when, in our view, it is not appropriate.[60] On other occasions, we fail to hear the word when the concept is in everyone's mind. Can the medical community achieve a consensus and put forward for public assessment a definition of medical futility? One answer is to point out that the courts will not await such a development but, rather, will continue to make ad hoc, emotionally propelled decisions,[61] or (as in the court-ordered treatment of an anencephalic baby) decisions based on idiosyncratic interpretations of federal statutes like the Americans with Disabilities Act, the Rehabilitation Act of 1973, and the Emergency Medical Treatment and Active Labor Act (enacted to prevent hospital "dumping"),[62] causing physicians and patients to become mired in ever more intractable confusion.

Therefore, the responsibility rests with the medical profession to take the initiative by offering specific standards and guidelines in the hope of first achieving consensus within the medical community and ultimately gaining acceptance in society at large. At the very least, hospitals should make clear to the public whether or not their futility policy is benefit-based or a "respectable alternative." The latter, for example, might specify the hospital's willingness to go along with family demands to maintain life-sustaining treatment on hospital-bound or permanently unconscious patients indefinitely. We have argued, however, that if this is a hospital's well-considered moral position rather than merely a vacuous nonposition, the hospital should be willing to act on its moral principle by accepting such patients as transfers from hospitals that have a benefit-based policy on futility.[63]

In summary, we call upon medical professionals to take the following steps:

1. Acknowledge that the word *futility* is widely used in medical practice and agree to use it in a more consistent and explicit fashion than it is today.

2. Seek a specific meaning for the concept through open debate and consensus-seeking. Start with the general proposal that medical futility means treatment that fails to achieve the goals of medicine, in that it offers no benefit to the patient above a minimal quantitative or qualitative threshold. Then see whether the medical profession can agree as to what counts as a minimum probability or minimal quality of benefit.

3. Introduce this definition of futility into practice by encouraging publication of studies reporting not only positive therapeutic outcomes (to be adopted) but also negative therapeutic outcomes (to be avoided). These empirical studies will form the basis for defining professional standards of care (also called practice guidelines) for clinical situations.

4. Seek to educate and obtain the concurrence of society at large by declaring these standards of care openly, as institutional policies for the information of the public (including legislatures and governmental agencies) and as guidelines for the courts.

CHAPTER TEN

The High Points

Medical Futility

In October 1992 a baby was born in a Virginia hospital with most of her brain, skull, and scalp missing—a condition called anencephaly. Because of this condition, which was recognized by ultrasound before birth, the baby, known as Baby K, was destined never to be conscious, able to think, see, hear, or otherwise interact with her environment. The physicians explained to Baby K's mother that the most they do for anencephalic infants is to blanket and hydrate them respectfully until they die, usually within a few days of birth. However, as soon as the newborn began to show signs of respiratory failure, the mother demanded all aggressive life-sustaining treatments, including mechanical ventilation and cardiopulmonary resuscitation if the heart stopped. Yielding to the mother's demands, the physicians did everything they could to keep Baby K alive.

After a month of this treatment, the hospital tried to transfer Baby K to another hospital more sympathetic to the mother's wishes; however, no hospital in the area would accept the infant, and the baby was instead placed in a bed in a nearby nursing home. Baby K died after two and a half years, after having been readmitted to the hospital repeatedly due to breathing difficulties. Each time, on the mother's insistence, the baby was given mechanical ventilation and other life-sustaining interventions, even though the physicians continued to argue that such treatments were inappropriate.

After attempts to resolve the matter through the hospital ethics committee failed, the hospital requested a court declaration that the hospital not be required to provide such treatments, arguing that "because of [anencephalic babies'] extremely limited life expectancy and because any treatment of their condition is futile," the standard of care is to provide comfort only.[1] However, in a series of court decisions rising to the level of the U.S. Court of Appeals for the Fourth Circuit, the mother's demands for continuing aggressive life-sustaining interventions were upheld.[2] The courts cited several federal statutes, claiming that refusal to treat Baby K would violate the Americans with Disabilities Act, the Rehabilitation Act of 1973, and the Emergency Medical Treatment and Active Labor Act (EMTALA, which was enacted solely to prevent hospitals from "dumping" patients who were unable to pay).[3]

This case exemplifies the vast gap between the goals of medicine and the strictures of the legal system. In particular, the language used by the courts in their analysis of the case illustrates the travesty that results from a failure to distinguish between an *effect* and a *benefit* of medical treatment.

For example, the court decisions (and even the amicus brief filed in support of the hospital by lawyers for the American Academy of Pediatrics and the Society of Critical Care Medicine) repeatedly referred to Baby K's "respiratory distress," a characterization that failed to recognize that the baby was incapable of experiencing any sensation, including distress. Placing the baby on a ventilator helped the lungs to pump air; however, the baby experienced no benefit from the effect of this treatment. Similarly, the Americans with Disabilities Act specifies: "No individual shall be discriminated against on the basis of disability in the full and equal enjoyment of the goods, services, facilities, privileges, advantages or accommodations."[4] Clearly, in using the term "enjoyment," Congress did not envisage application of this act to someone with no capacity to experience, much less enjoy.

The *Baby K* decision sent shudders throughout the health care system. A survey of neonatal pediatricians and ethics committee chairs at U.S. children's hospitals revealed disbelief, even outrage, at the decision, yet almost unanimous acknowledgement that they too would probably be forced by their hospital administration to do the same thing out of fears of litigation.[5] Ironically, in a later decision, the Fourth Circuit Court itself ruled that *Baby K* concerned only "stabilizing treatment that EMTALA required for a particular emergency medical condition. . . . EMTALA cannot plausibly be interpreted to regulate medical and ethical decisions outside [the emergency room] context."[6] Thus, the court explicitly limited application of the *Baby K* decision to the emergency room setting in order to stop hospitals from "dumping" indigent patients, and it reassured physicians that its ruling was not intended to interfere with general "medical and ethical decisions." Nevertheless, the decision has cast a shadow over many hospitals attempting to craft compassionate end-of-life treatment policies.

It probably should not be surprising during this time of soaring medical costs and proliferating technology that an intense debate has arisen over the notion of medical futility. Should doctors do all the things they are doing? In particular, should they attempt treatments that offer negligible likelihood of achieving the goals of medicine? What *are* the goals of medicine? Can we agree about what constitutes failure in such medical treatment? What should the physician do and not do under such circumstances? Exploring these issues forces us to revisit the doctor-patient relationship in a most fundamental way.[7]

Is There Such a Thing as Medical Futility?

If we look up the word *futility* in the *Oxford English Dictionary,* we learn that it means "leaky, vain, failing of the desired end through intrinsic defect." What then is the "failing of the desired end" in the case of medical futility? As we have pointed out in Chapter 1, some claim that the term *medical futility* has so many possible meanings that it is too elusive to define.[8]

One proposed definition of medical futility holds that futility should depend on the likelihood of achieving *the patient's goals.* In other words, the patient is entitled to demand any outcome he or she wishes from the physician, and the physician is not entitled to judge a treatment futile as long as it can offer something the patient wants. This view, which holds that the principle of respect for autonomy trumps every other principle or value in medicine, arose most forcefully during the 1960s, out of the patient-autonomy movement that developed in response to abuses that took place during the previous era of strong physician paternalism. And although the approach that puts autonomy front and center was a much-needed corrective to paternalism, it is not without flaws.

Physicians are *not* obligated to yield, for example, to a patient's desire for mutilating or useless surgery. As other bioethicists state: "The shift in emphasis from physicians' paternalism to the involvement of patients in the decision-making process is not a directive for physicians to abandon their judgment. Nor should it signal the elevation of patient autonomy to an absolute."[9] If the patient's goal is to become a world champion bodybuilder with the aid of steroids, the physician is neither ethically obligated nor legally permitted to comply with the bodybuilder's request. Nor is a surgeon obligated to perform a prophylactic appendectomy to assuage a patient's fears that her recurrent abdominal pains are due to appendicitis. These are but a few of the many instances of limitations and prohibitions on the physician's duty to achieve the patient's goal. A particularly important limitation, in this era of life-as-a-TV-movie-of-the-week, is that the physician does not owe the patient a miracle.

Another proposed definition of medical futility focuses on an unacceptable likelihood *of prolonging life*. Physicians, according to this position, cannot declare a treatment futile as long as it can prolong life, even permanently unconscious life. Those who make this claim are probably unaware that the obligation of physicians to prolong life is not supported by the classical tradition of medicine.[10] In ancient Greece and Rome, as expressed particularly through the Hippocratic writings, the physician's duties were described as assisting nature to restore health and alleviate suffering. Life and death were viewed as natural cycles; hence, any attempt to prolong life was not considered an appropriate goal of medicine. Indeed, the Hippocratic physician shunned claims of supernatural powers in order to avoid the taint of charlatanism. It was not until many centuries later, during the late Middle Ages, when religion began to play a dominant role in medical practice, and later in the seventeenth century, when scientists began to view science as a power to be exerted *against* nature, that the duty to prolong life was introduced. But it is important to keep in mind that neither theologians, nor scientists, nor for that matter anyone else before the modern era could ever have imagined life in the many forms it takes today—the many states between health and death that are the outcomes of modern medical treatments. Persistent vegetative state, to name just one condition describing the permanent unconsciousness of patients like Nancy Cruzan, Karen Ann Quinlan, and Terri Schiavo (now called permanent vegetative state), could not be found in medical textbooks nor was the term even coined until 1972.[11] Thus, the claim that the goal of medicine is to preserve life has ambiguous meanings and dubious roots in the historical tradition of the profession.

Another proposal limits the definition of medical futility to the unacceptable likelihood of achieving any *physiological effect* on the body. According to this proposal, the physician cannot regard a treatment as futile as long as it can maintain the function of any part of the body, such as pumping blood, digesting food, forming urine, or moving air, whether the patient is conscious or in the last moments of a terminal condition. This is sometimes presented as a "value-neutral" definition.[12] That there are those who seriously advocate this definition illustrates how much modern medicine has lost its way, how much it has become fragmented by subspecialties and technology. To choose narrow physiological criteria as the basis for the definition of medical futility is not "value-neutral," but a value *choice* that is, in our opinion, about as far from the patient-centered tradition of the medical profession as it is possible to be.

The definition of medical futility we support begins with the fundamental idea that medical interventions have as their goal helping the patient. Interventions with an unacceptably low likelihood or quality of therapeutic *benefit* for the *patient* are futile. Both italicized terms are important. A patient is neither a collection of organs nor merely an individual who has desires. Rather, a patient (from the word meaning "to suffer") is a person who seeks the healing (meaning "to make whole") powers of the physician. The relationship between effect and benefit is central to the healing process and the goals of medicine. The physician's charge is to provide not merely an *effect* on some part of the body but a *benefit* to the patient as a whole. Medicine today has the capacity to achieve a multitude of effects: raising and lowering blood pressure, speeding and slowing the heart, destroying cells, transplanting organs, to name but a few. But none of these effects is a benefit unless the patient has at the very least the capacity to appreciate it, a circumstance that is impossible if the patient is permanently unconscious, as in permanent vegetative state. Further, an effect is not a benefit if it cannot enable the patient to achieve at a minimum life goals other than complete "preoccupation" (to a use a term Plato attributed to the demigod-physician Asclepius) with the patient's illness and the treatment.

Medical Futility in Theory

The principle that physicians are not obligated to attempt futile treatment has not only existed throughout the history of medical practice but is endorsed today by a wide range of professional societies.[13] Lack of instant gratification with the short struggle to reach a definition of medical futility has caused some to plead that the term be abandoned altogether.[14] This is absurd. Medical futility is actively used in medical discourse for the very reason that it conveys a vital meaning in medical practice: some treatments fail to achieve the goals of medicine, and physicians are not obligated to attempt them. It is important that we make this clear to society as well as to the profession. Medicine has great powers but not unlimited powers. The medical profession has important obligations but not unlimited obligations. Failing to seek a precise meaning for the term only leaves us in a state of ambiguity that encourages the very abuses many people fear. Physicians should not be free to invoke medical futility unless they can justify it before their peers and before society. This requires that we examine the concept, not hide from it.

The Mythical Power of Medical Futility

As we have already seen, the ancient Greek *futtilis* was a religious vessel that had a wide top and a narrow bottom. This peculiar shape caused the vessel to tip over easily, which made it of no practical use for anything other than ceremonial occasions. The philosopher Don Postema has pointed out that in discussing futile treatment we should be aware that the root of the term reminds us that words have a mythical power as well as a literal meaning.[15] It is possible, therefore, that sometimes unrealistic expectations and unreasonable demands for futile treatments, such as attempted CPR in a cancer patient with barely hours to live, may be expressions of deep ritualistic needs. These actions in our modern time have become almost religious ceremonies. Indeed, it is not too extreme to point out that in the past, when patients sought a miracle, they went to church and prayed to God. Today they come to the hospital and demand it of the physician. Therefore, it is important to emphasize again: Physicians are not, and never were, obligated to produce a miracle.

What Futility Is Not

The word *futile* has to be distinguished from a variety of synonymic neighbors such as *impossible* (walking to the moon is not futile; it is impossible), *implausible* (producing a full-grown infant solely by in vitro techniques might be possible someday, but it is implausible today), and *rare* (in addition to rarity, futility carries an operational notion: success is rare, and therefore attempted treatment should not be obligatory). Nor is *futile* the equivalent *of hopeless.* Hope and hopelessness are psychological reactions to objective facts. Given our individual temperaments, if all of us happen to face the same small chance of success in a specific procedure, we are likely to experience different reactions, ranging from euphoric optimism to bleak pessimism. And although physicians regard hope as an important psychological aid in medical care, they should not invoke hope as justification for deceiving patients by misrepresenting the facts. There are better, more humane, ways to comfort patients.

Quantitative and Qualitative Medical Futility

As noted in Chapter 1, our definition of medical futility encompasses both quantitative and qualitative aspects. From the writings of the Hippocratic corpus we derived a quantitative aspect: "Whenever the illness is too strong for the available remedies, the physician surely must not expect that it can be overcome by medicine. . . . To attempt futile treatment is to display an ignorance that is allied to madness."[16] We can trace the qualitative aspect of medical futility back to the Platonic-Asclepian era. In Plato's *Republic* we find these statements: "For those whose lives are always in a state of inner sickness Asclepius did not attempt to prescribe a regime to make their life a prolonged misery. . . . A life of preoccupation with illness and neglect of work is not worth living."[17]

Quantitative Futility

The quantitative aspect of medical futility is tied to the uncertainty inherent in the practice of medicine. Every medical student learns to "never say never." And philosophers of science such as Karl Popper point out that even though one sees B follow A a hundred, or a thousand, or even a million, times, one can never be absolutely certain that the same thing will happen again. Nevertheless, as reasonable observers we inescapably begin to draw conclusions at some point in our observations. Similarly, if B has *never* followed A after many events, at some point we begin to draw conclusions about the likelihood that B will follow A, although again we can never be absolutely certain. This kind of commonsense empirical reasoning forms the basis for our daily living activities.

More particularly, it is the basis for the clinical practice of medicine. As one classic example, the effectiveness of vaccines to prevent diseases like hepatitis B and influenza is— like nearly every treatment—based on empirical observations. One cannot be absolutely certain the injection will prevent these diseases in every patient. Indeed, a rare patient develops a serious allergic reaction to the vaccine and almost certainly would be better off not having taken it. So to those who demand, "Are you absolutely certain?" the answer is always, "No." But that is not the correct question. Rather, the correct question is, How many times and to what degree do we have to fail before we agree to call a treatment futile?

In medicine, as in our daily affairs, we act on the basis of empirical evidence. To overcome the paralysis of uncertainty that may compel physicians to pursue even the most unlikely treatments, we propose what is nothing more than a commonsense definition of futility. Most of us probably would agree that if a treatment has not worked in the last 100 cases, it is almost certainly not going to work if it is tried again. (Statisticians can calculate that the upper limit of the 95% confidence interval is 3%.) This proposal is not an "objective" or "value-free" definition, but rather, one that seeks reasonable consensus where absolute certainty is impossible and therapeutic benefit is the goal. If we can agree to call such treatments futile, then the ordinary duty of the physician does not include offering them. The medical community, or society at large, may prefer longer (or shorter) odds, but in the end we all must accept some empirical notion of medical futility or throw common sense to the wind.

Is a consensus developing for medical futility? Interestingly, about the same time our original proposal was published in 1990,[18] researchers had already started to report empirical outcomes of life-saving treatments, ranging from the use of steroids in brain hemorrhage to cardiopulmonary resuscitation (CPR) in various clinical circumstances, including metastatic cancer and extreme prematurity.[19] In all the studies the researchers declared that when the treatment failed after a certain number of attempts, the treatment should be regarded as futile. What is striking is that the decision to call the treatment futile was made independently by these researchers (who were unaware at the time of one another's recommendations or of our proposed definition) after the number of failures fell within the same range we suggested in our original article. In other words, there appears to be a convergence of expert opinion in the medical community about a threshold for quantitative medical futility.

Qualitative Futility

The goal of medicine is not merely to provide an effect on the body; it is also to provide a benefit to the patient. Our contention, introduced in Chapter 1 and discussed throughout the book, is that a patient who is permanently un-conscious will never benefit from any treatment, being bereft of the capacity to appreciate any effect. Thus, any life-prolonging treatments provided for a patient in permanent vegetative state are by definition futile. We also referred to a notion attributed by Plato to Asclepius, that if the treatment fails to re-lease the patient from being "preoccupied" with the illness and incapable of achieving any other life goal, that treatment should also be regarded as futile. For example, if the only way physicians can keep a patient alive is by main-taining the patient on technology available only in an acute hospital setting, that outcome should not be regarded as a success. Rather, it is a failure to achieve the goals of medicine—which, at the very least, should be to restore the patient's health sufficiently to allow that person to survive outside the hospital. Such treatment, by our definition, is qualitatively futile.

Note that our outcome measure is consistent with that of researchers we cite above. They independently concluded that when life-saving treatments failed to result in survival to hospital discharge after a certain number of pa-tients were subjected to the treatment, then those treatments should be re-garded as futile. In our original publication we proposed a more restricted definition—namely, confinement to the intensive care unit. The evolution in our thinking is a good example of the stepwise manner in which consensus seeking must proceed. In the final analysis, the medical community and soci-ety at large must engage in critical reflection on both of these explicitly de-fined notions—escape from dependence on intensive care or discharge from the hospital (and others too, perhaps)—and decide which outcomes represent an ethical goal for medicine.

An Analogical Argument for Quantitative Medical Futility: The Placebo

In addition to a gathering empirical consensus, there is a strong analogi-cal argument supporting quantitative futility. Most of us are familiar with the powerful placebo effect of drugs, which in some studies are observed to be as high as 30 percent. Let us examine the implications of this phenome-non in the context of medical futility. If there were no limits to a physician's obligations—that is, if a physician were obligated to offer any treatment that may have worked in the past or that may conceivably work in the future—then in the absence of a proven treatment the physician would be ethically obligated to offer a placebo. But physicians are not ethically obligated to offer a placebo whenever a beneficial treatment is unavailable. There are, of course, good reasons for this. If patients knew that physicians were always going to prescribe *something*, there would be a complete breakdown of trust. Patients could never be sure when they were receiving a treatment specifically indicated for their condition and when they were receiving a placebo. Ironically, the benefit of the placebo effect of *all* drugs would probably vanish.

Ethical Implications and Physicians' Obligations

In addition to proposing a specific definition of futility in terms of the failure to achieve, at some minimal quantitative and qualitative thresholds, ethical goals of helping the patient, we also addressed (in Chapter 7) the question, What is the ethical obligation of the physician faced with a treatment that is futile?[20] We considered three possible answers to this question.

Physicians ought to be allowed to refrain from offering futile treatment but not be obligated to do so. Under this option, which we reject, the ethical implications for physicians would be analogous to therapeutic abortion. Abortion is ethically and legally permitted by society, but individual physicians are allowed to avoid offering it as a matter of personal moral choice. An important difference should be noted, however, between refusing to perform an abortion and claiming the right to keep a permanently unconscious patient alive indefinitely. In the former instance, the consequence of the physician's decision is limited to the patient, and that decision is unequivocally overridden by ethics and the law, which require that physician to refer the patient to a facility that will comply with the patient's legal request. In the latter instance, the physician's decision to continue treatment affects space, equipment, supplies, other patients, and a host of hospital workers. It has consequences for the entire institution. Therefore, we encourage health care institutions to develop futility policies or integrate such policies into existing policies governing withholding and withdrawal of treatment. Such policies should reflect input from physicians, nurses, and other health professionals, as well as the local community. Once policies are in place, individual physicians will not be allowed or expected to render futility judgments unilaterally, at the bedside, but will instead be held accountable to abide by institutional guidelines.

One of us (LJS) organized a conference in 1998 that involved 74 participants from 26 California hospitals, ranging from community hospitals to major university hospitals.[21] The purpose of the conference was to see whether a consensus on medical futility could be achieved. All but 2 of the hospitals had specific futility policies, and all but 2 of the 24 hospitals with such policies defined futile treatment in terms of benefit to the patient rather than physiological effect. This latter (majority) group of hospitals provides a basis for a definitional "majority standard." But there is still room for a "respectable minority," consistent with our pluralistic society. However, in our judgment, a "respectable minority" hospital that permits physicians to continue life-sustaining treatment on patients whose treatment other hospitals deem futile have taken an ethical position and should be willing to accept such patients in transfer. Certainly, this would spare the patient and loved ones of long, expensive, and emotionally draining court disputes.

Physicians ought to be encouraged to refrain from offering futile treatment but not be obligated to do so. Under this option, which we also reject, the ethical implications for physicians are analogous to maintaining patients in permanent vegetative state. Professional authorities have recommended against keeping such patients alive by medical means, but physicians are not obligated to follow such recommendations. As noted above, institutions that adhere to this standard would also qualify as operating under a "respectable minority" standard of care and should be willing to accept in transfer patients from "majority standard" hospitals.

Physicians should be obligated to refrain from offering futile treatment. Under this final option, which we defend in chapter 7 and throughout the book, the ethical implications for the physician would be analogous to treating patients with human immunodeficiency virus (HIV) infection. The medical profession has unequivocally imposed on its members the obligation to treat such patients. It is a declaration, not merely a recommendation, and physicians may not opt out because of personal moral objections alone. As noted above, the majority of California hospitals that participated in a statewide conference on medical futility have futility policies that accept this standard of care.[22]

Exceptions and Cautions

Although we seek to define and delineate the ethical implications of medical futility as precisely as possible, we recognize that medical practice calls on us to recognize certain exceptions and cautions.

If the physician is allowed, encouraged, or required to withhold a futile treatment, does this mean the physician enjoys the privilege of withholding discussion about such treatment? Certainly physicians do not describe to patients all the many tests and treatments they have no intention of pursuing. However, an important distinction exists between treatment and information. Depending on the context and the patient's state of mind, patients may be ethically entitled to information even if they are not entitled to treatments. In this regard, physicians should anticipate and recognize the concerns of patients within the particular context of medical care. A physician need not discuss the possibility of brain surgery with every patient who has a headache. On the other hand, any patient in the intensive care unit (ICU), looking around and seeing CPR attempted to the right and to the left (or on TV), is aware that this is one possible treatment option.

In such a setting, physicians owe their patients information and some discussion as to whether CPR should be attempted. Making a decision that a treatment is medically futile does not absolve the physician of the obligation to discuss and inform the patient about what is going on in terms of the patient's condition, prognosis, and treatment options. But it would be a mistake to create an exchange which in effect has the physician stating to the patient: "Attempting CPR would be of no use in treating your disease at this point. Do you want us to do it?" As other bioethicists point out, such a communication sends a meaningless, even contradictory, message that contributes to confusion and distrust on the part of the patient.[23] Rather than assisting the patient in exercising autonomy, it actually deceives the patient and prevents full exercise of autonomy.

What about the terminally ill patient who requests attempted CPR to allow one last visit from a distant loved one who is hastening to the bedside? Even though the physician is convinced that CPR has almost no chance of keeping the patient alive more than a day or so in the ICU, clearly the physician will want to make an exception to accommodate the short-term goal of the patient. It is important, however, to distinguish this limited, compassionate act from an open-ended, obligatory act. The physician can easily make a compassionate exception in the case of a severely burned patient or a patient with metastatic cancer whose request for treatment will result in a small extension of life (a clear and limited goal and a small exception to the physician's duty). But in the case of permanent vegetative state, obligating the physician to accede to a request for long-term life-prolongation could lead to decades of futile treatment. Contrary to those who raise fears that a recognition of medical futility devalues the patient, giving the physician the opportunity to view each patient as a unique person in unique circumstances *enhances* the value of the individual and encourages the use of appropriate medical measures rather than the useless, thoughtless pursuit of inappropriate measures.

The Importance of Defining Medical Futility

During the early stages of any controversial debate, people may feel tempted to push the problem they are dealing with out of sight.[24] There is an important heuristic value to the search for a clear definition of medical futility, whatever definition emerges.[25]

First of all, the futility debate has already resulted in more clarity of thinking, particularly in distinguishing medical futility from rationing. As discussed at length in Chapter 5, medical futility signifies that a treatment offers no therapeutic benefit to the individual patient. Rationing specifically acknowledges that a treatment *does* offer a benefit, and the issue becomes how to distribute limited resources fairly among the many patients who stand to benefit. With rationing, the central concern is establishing ethical criteria and priorities to apply to medically qualified patients.[26]

Oregon was one of the first states to address these kinds of rationing questions in developing a policy for its Medicaid program, a public program designed to provide health care coverage to the poor. In the original Oregon plan, however, some of the treatments that were below the funding cut-off line actually represented futile treatments: they offered patients no therapeutic benefit. These treatments do not strictly qualify under the category of rationing because no matter how cheap or available such treatments are, there is no point in attempting them. On the other hand, rationing decisions do have to be made about treatments such as heart transplants, renal dialysis, and other expensive and otherwise restricted treatments because they offer clear-cut benefits to patients in need of these treatments. To clarify further the distinction: Futility decisions are made at the bedside of a specific patient, whereas rationing decisions, involving categories of patients or treatments or circumstances, inevitably should be made at a policy level in order to assure just distribution of resources.

A second value to pursuing a clear-cut concept of medical futility is that doing so encourages a more aggressive search for precisely the kind of information that our medical enthusiasm has caused us to overlook. We refer to the publication of clinical trials and retrospective studies that report not only treatments that are successful, but also treatments that are *not* successful. This is what is meant by "evidence-based medicine." Both kinds of data are important to the practice of medicine; both provide guidelines for physician and societal choice.

Third, pursuing a clear concept of medical futility will oblige us to see whether or not the medical profession can achieve consensus, one that is also acceptable to society. As we have already noted, there seems to be evidence that a consensus about quantitative futility exists and is growing throughout the medical community. It was just this process of medical attention to an important ethical issue that led to today's Uniform Definition of Death Act.

Beyond Futility to an Ethic of Care

In this second edition of *Wrong Medicine*, we reiterate our concerns that those who adamantly oppose the concept of medical futility focus too narrowly on whether to employ particular life-saving medical treatments.[27] This has caused the neglect of an important area: the physician's obligation to alleviate suffering, enhance well-being, and support the dignity of the patient in the last few days of life. We urge that discussions, both in public and at the bedside, be expanded beyond "pull-the-plug" decisions to include more vigorous attention to improving doctor-nurse interactions, so that doctors who have "nothing to offer" do not walk away leaving to nurses the "nursing care"—seemingly beneath the physicians' attention. Patients and families who demand "Do everything!" may well be expressing a subtext: "Do not abandon me!"

We also call on health care professionals to continue the process that is already under way: persuading our institutions to set aside rooms and areas enabling family members to gather around a dying patient in a setting that maximizes intimacy and dignity as opposed to the dehumanized, efficiency-oriented areas that characterize most ICUs today.

Finally, we hope that any new developments in national health care reform will not only generously reimburse the cost of comfort and palliative care, whether in the home or the hospice setting, but also send a strong message to physicians that comfort care is an expected, valued part of caring for patients at the end of life.[28] Sadly, as we witnessed in congressional health care debates during the Obama administration, many politicians and religious extremists have misrepresented and scorned attempts to promote humane care at the end of life, scurrilously attacking the proposal to offer Medicare reimbursement for physicians who consult with patients on end-of-life planning as government-mandated "death panels."

Evidence suggests that much work lies ahead. Two recent articles reported that elderly nursing home patients were receiving futile treatments in place of more appropriate end-of-life counseling and support. In one study that looked at the health records of 3,702 nursing home residents nationwide who started dialysis, there was a marked decline in functional status during the period surrounding the initiation of dialysis. The residents—whose average age was 73 and who often had other serious health problems in addition to failing kidneys, such as diabetes, heart disease, and cancer—were not benefiting from the dialysis treatment they were receiving. The authors concluded that physicians should not automatically begin dialysis in this population and should instead target "efforts to address the goals of care, alleviate suffering, and maintain functional independence."[29]

Another study of elderly nursing home residents who had advanced dementia reported that these residents experience a high mortality rate, with death often preceded by infections, eating problems, and distressing symptoms. The authors found that within this population during the three months before death many residents "underwent burdensome interventions of questionable benefit." At the same time the authors noted that "when health care proxies were aware of the poor prognosis and the expected clinical complications, residents were less likely to undergo these interventions in the final days of life." The authors conclude, on the basis of their own evidence and multiple studies from the medical literature, that the life expectancy for patients who have advanced dementia is comparable to the life expectancy of patients who have terminal illnesses, such as metastatic breast cancer and class IV (the most severe) congestive heart failure: "The idea that dementia is a terminal illness is further supported by our findings that most of the deaths were not precipitated by devastating acute events (e.g., myocardial infarction), other terminal diseases (e.g., cancer), or the decompensation of chronic conditions (e.g., congestive heart failure)."[30]

We concur with these authors that doctors and families should make the feeble and cognitively impaired elderly patients who are near death comfortable, rather than treating them as if cure is possible.

Our proposal will require not only changing medical practice and reforming the reimbursement for medical services, but also engaging and educating the public about the concepts and realities of medical futility, along with the ethical goals of medicine.

Distinguishing Treatment from Experiment

Following the arguments we present here and in the earlier (1995) edition of this book, it is evident that once a treatment is shown to be futile, it should no longer be offered to patients. Where uncertainty exists about whether or not a treatment will benefit a group of patients, treatment can be ethically offered, but only in the context of an experimental trial, which requires a reasonable hypothesis, Institutional Review Board approval, and informed consent that acknowledges that the patient is participating in an experiment rather than a treatment. For example, now that attempted CPR in hospitalized and bed-bound patients with metastatic cancer is known to be futile, that intervention should not be offered. Continuing to shock, pound, and pump patients' chests in this situation does not benefit them and is not ethically supported. Moreover, choosing to attempt CPR in such a situation allows medicine to evade its responsibility to look for better alternatives and move forward. In this situation, either new techniques or more precise indications should be established as promising hypotheses before attempting CPR, or alternatively, more clearly defined policies emphasizing comfort care should be put in place.

Patients' Rights to Unproven Treatments

From the arguments presented here it should also be clear that we oppose claims that patients have a right to any treatment they wish if their disease is serious and no treatment of proven benefit is available. Activists for cancer and Alzheimer's disease have sometimes used this argument to persuade the Food and Drug Administration to change its approval policy from one of protecting the unwitting consumer to one of expediting drugs on a treatment basis before they are shown to be beneficial. Although we sympathize with patients and loved ones who feel desperate about overcoming a poor prognosis, we also recognize a responsibility to avoid harming patients: multitudes of patients inevitably suffer as a consequence of this revised policy. Sanctioning dubious drugs before their therapeutic efficacy is established by careful clinical trials only *delays* the discovery of useful drugs because it makes recruitment of patients into prospective clinical trials more difficult. Unfortunately, only a rare drug turns out to fulfill its early promise. Thus many patients, deceived into thinking that drugs provided under medical auspices must be beneficial, are actually more likely to experience harmful side effects without compensating benefits.

CHAPTER ELEVEN

Medical Futility

Where Do We Stand Now?

In our original journal article on medical futility, before the publication of the first edition of *Wrong Medicine*, the two of us, along with our colleague the philosopher and bioethicist Albert R. Jonsen, introduced a definition of medical futility and discussed its ethical implications.[1] We realized that although the concept had been acknowledged and respected even before the time of Hippocrates, it suddenly seemed new and controversial to many of today's practitioners, trained in age of high-technology medicine. In our article we said, "We recognize—indeed invite—examination and challenge of our proposal." Since then and since the book's publication in 1995, the three of us have responded to a number of critiques of the concept of medical futility.[2] In this final chapter, "Medical Futility: Where Do We Stand Now," we use the word "stand" with two meanings: Where do we stand now, meaning what is the current status of medical futility in the health care community? And where do we stand now, meaning what is our current opinion of the concept of medical futility? In the following pages we summarize the major objections we have encountered and our responses. We offer these here so that you, the reader, have an opportunity to evaluate these exchanges and consider where *you* stand.

Objections and Responses

Objection 1: Medical futility is an attempt to increase the power of the physician over the patient and repeal recent hard-gained advances in patient autonomy.

The basic premise underlying this argument is that the physician and the patient are inexorably locked in "a war between doctor and patient over who gets to decide what."[3] In this power struggle, the physician (who has little to lose) possesses expert knowledge and control over technology. By contrast, the patient, whose life may hang in the balance, typically possesses little expert knowledge and no authority over technological interventions.[4] Those who make this argument hold that endorsing the physician's power to declare a treatment futile gives the physician a "trump card" or a "conversation stopper" that interferes with the meager power the patient retains (the power of persuasion) in the physician-patient dialogue.[5] We and others have pointed out, however, that the power to make judgments about futility is a necessary part of the physician's duty of beneficence, that is, the duty to use only treatments that provide therapeutic benefits.[6] This power resides not with the individual physician's arbitrary whim, but with the profession as a whole as it establishes general standards of care based on the best available evidence. In our view, abuses of power are resolved, not by eliminating medical judgment and yielding to unreasonable demands, but rather by exercising judgment openly and responsibly according to professional standards.[7]

Clearly, some wishes and needs are beyond the scope of informed consent and exceed the limits of the physician's obligation. For example, a physician treating a patient for severe depression might conclude that if the patient could only get his or her finances in order, the patient would be much less depressed. The physician might be sympathetic to the patient's distress and might even try to recommend help, but surely no one would claim that balancing the patient's bank account is an obligatory medical duty. Physicians are more often under pressure to use the vast array of technologies at their disposal when those technologies may keep organ systems functioning even though the patient is no longer able to appreciate any benefit from these interventions. Means are confused with ends, effects are confused with benefits, and available technologies are confused with obligatory medical therapies. In our experience, requests for futile treatment often represent not an appeal to respect the patient's wishes,[8] but rather a misguided effort to express caring for the patient by meeting a perceived duty to "do everything" when other manifestations of devotion (such as comfort care) would be wiser and more appropriate.[9] Or they represent the failure, on the part of patients, families, and health professionals, to face and accept the inevitability of death as the final chapter of a human life.

Objection 2: No professional or societal consensus has been achieved about the definition of futility.

Impatience with the slow pace of resolving such a complex ethical issue has led some critics to conclude that efforts to define and apply "futility" are themselves futile.[10] Studies have shown that physicians disagree about quantitative and qualitative thresholds for futility.[11]

However, persons with long experience in public opinion research point out that achieving consensus is a gradual and evolving process. It begins with public awareness of an issue, proceeds to understanding by working through the issue (which, in the case of medical futility, will require changing unrealistic expectations about what medicine and science can accomplish), and finally leads to resolution on cognitive, emotional, and moral levels.[12] It is worth remembering that achieving nationwide consensus on a universal definition of death according to whole-brain criteria took approximately 20 years. Compared with this, the futility debate is still in its adolescence.

To those who are concerned that the medical profession is seeking to impose its own notion of futility on the public,[13] we emphasize that every profession declares values and standards. In the case of health care, the various professions should present their values openly and repeatedly to society by advancing the standards of practice and then subjecting these values to the scrutiny of legislatures and courts.[14] Acting through legislative, licensing, and court decisions, society accepts or rejects professional standards.

In the past several years, hospitals, state legislatures, and working groups of professionals and laypersons have developed consensus-based futility policies. (See Chapter 3.) At the professional level, the American Medical Association issued a Code of Medical Ethics in 1996 declaring that "all health care institutions, whether large or small, should adopt a policy on medical futility." The AMA further stated that policies on medical futility should follow "due process in specific cases," starting with earnest attempts to deliberate and negoti-ate what constitutes futile treatment and what falls within acceptable limits for the physician, the family and the institution. The organization also con-cluded that if transfer to an institution whose policies allow futile treatment "is not possible, the intervention need not be offered" by institutions that do have limits. Later, in 2009, the AMA expanded on its earlier declaration by seeking congressional legislation "that will allow the creation of a methodol-ogy directed by physicians (MDs/DOs) that permits physicians (MD/DOs) to either not engage in or to suspend futile care at the end of life," and asked that physicians be legally protected from liability when "such decisions are made in good faith and within the standard of care with clear and convincing legal and ethical standards."

At the state legislative level, Texas passed an Advance Directives Act in 1999 that sets out specific steps to resolve disagreements before withdrawal of futile treatment. In the end, if the dispute is not resolved and if after 10 days of searching no other hospital can be located that will accept the patient, and if a judge determines there is no reasonable likelihood of finding a willing provider of the disputed treatment, the treatment "may be unilaterally with-drawn by the treatment team with immunity from civil and criminal prosecu-tion."[15] This "legal safe harbor" for physicians, institutions, and ethics com-mittees is the first of its kind in the country.

At the federal level, the Uniform Health-Care Decisions Act (1994) states: "A health care provider or institution may decline to comply with an indi-vidual instruction or health care decision that requires medically ineffective health care or health care contrary to generally accepted health care standards applicable to the health care provider or institution."[16] It further clarifies that "medically ineffective" health care means "treatment which would not offer the patient any significant benefit."[17] This statute has already been adopted by more than a half dozen states. These events suggest that the profession and society are already in the process of examining, understanding, and resolving issues of medical futility.

Objection 3: Futility is a value-laden determination whose use by medicine is inappropriate unless one sticks to a so-called value-free or strict physiologic definition of futility.

Some critics insist that only a narrow physiologic definition of medical fu-tility is ethically defensible because only a narrow definition is "value-free," although they do not agree on what constitutes "physiologic futility."[18] Contrary to the assertion that physiologic futility is value-free, we argue that it entails a *value choice*. Specifically, it assumes that the goals of medicine are to preserve organ function, body parts, and physiologic activity—an assumption that departs dramatically from the patient-centered goals of medicine.[19] Indeed, as we noted in Chapter 9, this confusion between effects and benefits can be viewed as part of the generic confusion of focusing on (and drawing erroneous conclusions from) surrogate laboratory measures (e.g., red blood cells or glucose) rather than on patient outcomes (namely, cardiovascular and diabetic mortality). This narrow focus can cause physicians to misjudge the value of treatment.[20]

Objection 4: Medical futility is a useless concept because empirical treatment data cannot be applied with certainty to any given patient.

It is sometimes argued that no matter how much data researchers assemble about a group of patients, the physician cannot be absolutely certain that the data apply to a particular case with its own unique clinical variables.[21] However, as the philosopher Karl Popper pointed out, "The old scientific ideal of episteme—of absolutely certain, demonstrable knowledge—has proved to be an idol. The demand for scientific objectivity makes it inevitable that every scientific statement must remain tentative for ever. It may indeed be corroborated, but every corroboration is relative to other statements which, again, are tentative. Only in our subjective experiences of conviction, in our subjective faith, can we be 'absolutely certain.'"[22]

This explains why the judgment of experienced clinicians will always be essential to rendering judgments of futility. Yet such judgments are, in this respect, no different from other medical judgments that require the application of clinical data to a particular patient. For example, in the treatment of congestive heart failure, the drugs, doses, and schedules to be prescribed to a particular patient are determined by using data collected from large samples of other patients. The experienced physician knows that one can never be certain that every patient will have the same response; therefore, the physician does not merely pigeonhole the case "without consideration of [the patient's] individual clinical circumstances."[23] However, the physician must start somewhere, namely with empirical experience. As we have noted (Chapter 1), such empirical experience has already been collected and used to provide standards of withholding attempted out-of-hospital CPR according to the proposal we made for determining quantitative futility in our published definition of medical futility.[24] In contrast to experimental treatments, for which evidence may be promising but insufficient, futile treatments have empirically failed to show a significant likelihood or quality of benefit.[25]

Some have argued that our quantitative threshold for futility is "arbitrary" and "without defense."[26] In fact, our defense is the same as the justification used in the statistical evaluation of clinical trials. This justification procedure compares treatment observations against the null hypothesis (no difference) in light of the conclusion that these observations have a 1 in 20 chance of being nonsignificant ($p = 0.05$) or, more conservatively, a 1 in 100 chance of being nonsignificant ($p = 0.01$). In other words, one can never be certain, even in large-scale studies, that a treatment is beneficial (better than no treatment or an alternative treatment); therefore, one submits observations to the test of reasonableness. The notion of reasonableness is accepted in another major sector of society where a person's life may be at stake: courts of law. A jury in a criminal trial may find a defendant guilty and subject to the death penalty if the evidence is persuasive beyond a *reasonable* doubt, not beyond all doubt.

Thus, the proper question to ask is not whether we can be certain a treatment will not work but how many times we are willing to see a treatment fail before we agree that it does not work.[27] Contrary to the claim that our quantitative threshold provides "an illusion of objectivity,"[28] we have proposed that a standard of success in fewer than 1 in 100 cases is reasonable. The experience of 100 cases is attainable in many areas of medicine. Some may prefer a higher or lower standard or different standards for different clinical circumstances, but a line must be drawn somewhere short of "absolute certainty."

In contrast to our proposal, the American Heart Association guidelines for CPR and emergency cardiac care declared that treatments should be considered futile only if "no survivors after CPR have been reported under the given circumstances in well-designed studies."[29] Yet, as we argued in Chapter 9, this guideline failed to provide a quantitative threshold indicating at what point one can conclude that there are "no survivors." The American Heart Association also did not indicate whether "well-designed studies" should include dozens, hundreds, thousands, or even millions of participants.[30] Similarly, Prendergast, after objecting to the threshold we propose, goes on to say that "autonomy does not require physician compliance with a patient request where the evidence shows no benefit. Where the evidence is clear and convincing, autonomy is irrelevant."[31] However, Prendergast failed to identify the threshold that he uses to define "clear and convincing."

Finally, we note that the few studies (published by investigators who were unaware of each other's conclusions) that recommend that a treatment no longer be attempted because of its futility show a consensus of about the same magnitude as our original proposal.[32] Although skeptics doubt that a consensus will ever be reached, we find that professional agreement about medical futility seems already to be emerging. A good example is the publication of a Basic Life Support guideline based on empirical outcomes and subjected to the reasonable quantitative recommendation we proposed.[33]

Admittedly and unsurprisingly, the number of published studies that describe futile interventions is sparse when compared with the vast literature that describes successful interventions. Researchers always prefer to publish positive results. This does not mean that such studies are not being done. In fact, data on negative clinical outcomes are being assembled by managed health care organizations and health insurance providers, and these findings are beginning to challenge the efficacy (and more particularly the cost) of many traditional treatments. Some politicians have reacted to these efforts by raising the scary "R" word—rationing—as though irrational rationing, including the costly application of vastly overpriced (because useless) treatments, does not already exist. And sadly, the reaction of many medical professionals also has been to resist these perceived invasions of their freedom. This is unconscionable. In our opinion, the profession should assume far more responsibility in gathering these data.[34]

An exception is the important work done by medical investigators to characterize the prognosis of patients in various clinical circumstances.[35] Some critics argue that few futile treatments can confidently be said to have less than a 1 in 100 chance of success.[36] We see this as a stimulus to further research. Not only do we encourage continuous development and refinement of scoring systems; we also point out that scoring systems are not the only guides for experienced clinicians. Some clinical conditions can be characterized without a quantitative index. For example, certain congenital malformations, chromosomal abnormalities, neurologic degenerations, and advanced pulmonary diseases have never been reversed. Their anatomical character precludes treatment benefit. At a certain point in the clinical course of disease (sometimes very early, sometimes much later), most physicians recognize that a treatment is futile according to professional standards of care.

Objection 5: Medical futility undermines our pluralistic society and threatens, among other things, the free exercise of religion.

Some maintain that religious and medical goals are inextricably intertwined and therefore that medical futility interferes with the free exercise of religion. Post argues that approximately one-fifth of the text in the New Testament gospels describes the healing of physical or mental illness and the resurrection of the dead and that "even in mainstream Protestant churches, the belief in miraculous healing exists."[37]

Post's argument persuades us that religion and contemporary Western medicine should be regarded as independent activities that seek the goal of healing in different ways. In the gospel stories, healing is usually achieved not through medical treatments but by the laying on of hands, so that "the blind see, the lame walk, the lepers are cleansed, the deaf hear, [and] the dead are raised" (Luke 7:22). Physicians are mentioned only in a description of how they failed to heal "a woman having an issue of blood twelve years, which had spent all her living on physicians, neither could be healed of any." The woman's bleeding was immediately staunched by touching the border of Jesus's garment (Luke 8:43-44). By contrast, medical practitioners have been forced to acknowledge the limits of their art since the time of Hippocrates. Medicine, according to gospel teachings, cannot be expected to respond to the farthest reaches of religion; there, revelation, faith, and miraculous healing (including the restoration of life to the dead) are invoked. Miracles may be an important goal of prayer for many patients, but they should not be imposed on physicians as a goal of medical practice. Indeed, the very meaning of "miracle" depends on the premise that "the things which are impossible with men are possible with God" (Luke 18:27).

We have no objections when patients, families, and members of a religious faith choose to engage in meaningful religious and cultural activities; indeed, we respectfully encourage these actions. However, just as educators in the United States are not obligated to teach creationism in response to religious fundamentalists, western medical practitioners should not be expected to act contrary to personal or professional practice standards in response to persons who seek divine cures.[38]

As we have pointed out, our proposal provides a basis for a definitional "majority standard" of practice for U.S. hospitals. And although after reading this book you should be in no doubt how strongly we support this majority standard, this does not mean we wish to impose it as an arbitrary rule for all medical institutions. On the contrary, we maintain that there is room in this country for "respectable minority" hospitals that for whatever well-considered reasons, including religious ones, choose to permit physicians to continue life-sustaining treatments other hospitals deem futile. Accepting this respectable alternative standard would be consistent with our pluralistic society. We recognize that Catholic hospitals can refuse to perform a legal abortion—as long as they refer patients seeking that procedure to a "majority standard" hospital. However, as we have argued in previous chapters, if a "respectable minority" hospital has taken an ethical position and not merely a vacuous nonposition on medical futility—for example, endorsing life-sustaining treatment in a permanently unconscious patient—it should be willing to live up to its principled position and accept such patients in transfer from a "majority standard" hospital. As we have pointed out, this would spare the family long, expensive, and emotionally draining court trials.

Objection 6: Because rationing and resource allocation will ultimately determine medical futility, medical futility is an unnecessary concept.

Some critics predict that the futility debate will inevitably be submerged in the onrushing debate about limited money and resources.[39] We have discussed elsewhere (Chapter 5) the distinctions between futile and rationed treatments and between medical and societal justice.[40] In summary, rationing refers to the allocation of beneficial treatments among patients; futility refers to whether a treatment will benefit an individual patient. Although physicians have limited ethical authority to allocate finite medical resources on the basis of medical benefits to patients, only society has the ethical mandate to decide the relevance of nonmedical criteria in the allocation of scarce resources.

Clearly, we do not endorse the use of futility by physicians as a false cover for cost-containment strategies.[41] Such deception makes a mockery of the physician's assertion of professional integrity. Yet if the medical profession retreats to the position that it has no internal professional values and merely provides whatever patients, families, or insurers are willing to pay for, it can no longer claim to be a healing profession—that is, a group committed to helping and serving the sick. Instead, medicine becomes a commercial enterprise, not unlike the "oldest profession," whose sole purpose becomes satisfying the desires of others.

Critics who urge that the "rapid advance of the language of futility should be followed by an equally rapid retreat"[42] would dispose of a concept that has been intrinsic to medical practice since the time of Hippocrates, when the physician was mandated to "refuse to treat those who are overmastered by their diseases, realizing that in such cases medicine is powerless."[43] Simply put, medicine cannot always achieve its desired goals.[44] We urge the medical profession not to banish the "language of futility" but to examine that language more deeply and to look at the roots of the practice embedded in that language. Words that are central to health care, such as *heal* ("to make whole") and *patient* (from the Latin "to suffer"), suggest that the goal of medicine is not merely to achieve a means, such as restoring heartbeat, unless that means leads to the end of healing the patient.[45] At the same time, we acknowledge that in conversations with patients and families, it is crucial to show sensitivity and give assurance that the patient will not be abandoned, and that everything possible will be done to maintain the patient's comfort and dignity. Futility should not be deployed as a conversation stopper, but should instead be used in the context of a positive conversation about how the physicians and team can help the patient.

The Next Steps

What are the next steps going forward? First, we should all acknowledge that medical futility is not something that can be dismissed from the discourse of health care. It has a substantive meaning and plays an important role in pointing to the goals and limits of medicine. It is widely used, and so we urge that it be used with clarity and accountability. The challenge is to use the term in a clear and consistent fashion, and in a manner that reflects the goals of medicine. Abuses are more likely to occur in settings where institutional policies governing futility are vague or absent. Left without such a standard, physicians may invoke the term *futility* for a variety of unjustifiable reasons, ranging from a fear of being exposed to life-threatening infection, to avoiding patients they find distasteful, to an objection to providing costly therapies.[46]

Second, physicians and other health professionals should lead the way in futility debates by investigating and publishing studies that report not only positive therapeutic outcomes (to be adopted) but also negative therapeutic outcomes (to be avoided). Medical practice requires knowledge not only of what works but also of what doesn't work. An encouraging sign in recent health care reform efforts (enacted over the objection of confused politicians and profit-minded suppliers of drugs and devices) is the inclusion of funding for "effectiveness research."

Third, we invite future inquiries, in the form of books and articles like this one that will provide the stimulus for the medical profession and the community at large to engage in education and open debate. We propose a *patient-centered* account of medical futility, which defines a futile treatment as one that offers no benefit to the patient above a minimum quantitative and qualitative threshold. Then comes the fine tuning: can the medical profession, and ultimately society, agree about where to draw the line at a minimum probability or minimum quality of benefit? In other words, how many times and to what degree should we have to fail before we agree to call a treatment futile?

Fourth, we encourage continuing empirical studies as well as consensus agreements that form the basis for establishing professional standards of care. These standards of care should be declared openly as institutional policies by medical centers and organizations of medicine for the information of the public and as guidelines to the court. This last point is extremely important. Right now, as we have warned, many physicians still practice and many patients still receive treatment in an environment where ad hoc and often capricious decisions are rendered according to no agreed standards. Patients and patients' families are sometimes forced to pay for inhumane, unwanted care either because of an individual physician's misguided notions of medical duty or as a result of hasty, ill-conceived court decisions. Many physicians admit that they practice "defensive medicine," fearing that anything less than mindless continuation of aggressive treatments would make them legally vulnerable. As a consequence, they give the courts little guidance but to "do everything possible."

We hope that the debate over medical futility will encourage a revisiting of the doctor-patient relationship and will foster a more realistic understanding of the powers and limits of medicine. We hope that it will also bring into better synchrony the desires of patients, the hopes of families, and the ethical ends of medicine.[47]

Notes

CHAPTER ONE: Are Doctors Supposed to Be Doing This?

1. *Cruzan v. Director, Missouri Department of Health*, 110 S. Ct. 2841 (1990).
2. Multi-Society Task Force on Persistent Vegetative State, "Medical Aspects of the Persistent Vegetative State," *New England Journal of Medicine* 330 (1994): 1499–1508, 1572–79. This document provides a comprehensive update and recommends distinctions in terminology. The task force defines the vegetative state as "a condition of complete unawareness of the self and the environment accompanied by sleep-wake cycles with either complete or partial preservation of hypothalamic and brain stem autonomic functions." The task force distinguishes between the diagnostic entity *persistent* vegetative state, which refers to the clinical condition if it persists for at least one month, and *permanent* vegetative state, which carries prognostic implications of irreversibility. Permanent vegetative state is "an irreversible state, a definition, as with all clinical diagnoses in medicine, based on probabilities, not absolutes." The task force states that a patient in a persistent vegetative state "becomes permanently vegetative when the diagnosis of irreversibility can be established with a high degree of clinical certainty, i.e., when the chance of regaining consciousness is exceedingly rare." Throughout this book, we will refer to the vegetative state in terms that are consistent with the task force's recommendations.

More recently, researchers discovered that a few patients clinically diagnosed as permanently or minimally unconscious had areas of brain activity detected by functional magnetic resonance imaging (fMRI) when prompted to perform mental imagery tasks like hitting a tennis ball or walking inside their house. M. M. Monti, A. Vanhaudenhuyse, M. R. Coleman, et al., "Willful Modulation of Brain Activity in Disorders of Consciousness," *New England Journal of Medicine*, accessed February 3, 2010. In an accompanying editorial, Allan H. Ropper comments that "although this activation is surprising, it does not necessarily reveal conscious experience." Ropper goes on to point out: "Research on clinically undetected consciousness is easily subject to overinterpretation and sensationalism. . . . First, in this study, brain activation was detected in very few patients. Second, activation was found only in some patients with traumatic brain injury, not in patients with global ischemia and anoxia [such as following cardiac arrest]. Third, cortical activation does not provide evidence of an internal 'stream of thought' (William James's term), memory, self-awareness, reflection, synthesis of experience, symbolic representations, or—just as important—anxiety, despair, or awareness of one's predicament. Without judging the quality of any person's inner life, we cannot be certain whether we are interacting with a sentient, much less a competent, person. Moreover, persons who look to this study to justify continued and unqualified life support in all unresponsive patients are missing the focus of the findings." A. H. Ropper, "Cogito Ergo Sum by MRI," *New England Journal of Medicine*, accessed February 3, 2010.

3. *Cruzan v. Harmon*, 760 S.W. 2d 408 (Mo. 1988), *cert. granted sub nom.; Cruzan v. Director, Missouri Dept. of Health et al.*, 106 L. Ed. 2d 587, 109 S. Ct. 3240 (1989).

4. *In re Torres*, 357 N.W. 2d 341 (Minn. 1984). Years later, in 2001, the California Supreme Court copied *its* definition of "clear and convincing" from a previous Michigan decision, *In re Martin*, 538 N.W. 2d 399, 411 (Mich. 1995): "Only when the patient's prior statements clearly illustrate a serious, well thought out, consistent decision to refuse treatment under these exact circumstances, or circumstances highly similar to the current situation, should treatment be refused or withdrawn." *Conservatorship of Wendland*, 26 Cal. 4th 519 (2001), no. S087265. As can be seen from the language, both courts were oblivious to how little foresight laypersons have to anticipate their "exact circumstances" at the end of life.

5. *Cruzan v. Harmon*, 760 S.W. 2d 408 (Mo. 1988), *cert. granted sub nom.; Cruzan*, 106 L. Ed. 2d 587.

6. J. Cruzan, personal communication.

7. G. J. Annas, "The Long Dying of Nancy Cruzan," *Law, Medicine, and Health Care* 19 (1991): 52–59.

8. Multi-Society Task Force on Persistent Vegetative State, "Medical Aspects of the Persistent Vegetative State"; J. L. Bernat, *Ethical Issues in Neurology*, 3rd ed. (Philadelphia: Lippincott Williams & Wilkins, 2008), p. 295; S. Haidinger and G. Binder, "Prevalence of Persistent Vegetative State/Apallic Syndrome in Vienna," *European Journal of Neurology* 11 (2004): 461–66; J. C. Lavrisjen, J. S. van den Bosch, R. T. Koopmans, and C. van Weel, "Prevalence and Characteristics of Patients in a Vegetative State in Dutch Nursing Homes," *Journal of Neurology, Neurosurgery, and Psychiatry* 76 (2005): 1420–24.

9. Some observers attribute the change in attitude to a technological advance, namely, the introduction of percutaneous endoscopic gastrostomy (placing the feeding tube through the abdominal wall directly into the stomach). This procedure can be carried out easily under local anesthesia and is more comfortable for the patient. However, this causal argument is not persuasive, because patients in permanent vegetative state are incapable of feeling pain or the removal of any tube and could have been readily kept alive by being fed through a nasogastric tube. It is more likely that the attitude and the technology evolved concurrently and interdependently.

10. For a while, terms such as *irreversible coma, cerebral death, irreversible cessation of cerebral function,* and *coma dépassé* were used to describe the ambiguous state between permanent unconsciousness and death that presented in a patient whose electroencephalogram (EEG) showed no evidence of cerebral activity. Interestingly, despite the absence of universal agreement on criteria for withdrawing mechanical aids to respiration and circulation, the *Journal of the American Medical Association* was able to report in 1969 that "no one has encountered any medicolegal difficulties. Very few have sought legal opinions." D. Silverman, M. G. Saunders, R. S. Schwab, and R. L. Masland, "Cerebral Death and the Electroencephalogram: Report of the Ad Hoc Committee of the American Electroencephalographic Society on EEG Criteria for Determination of Cerebral Death," *JAMA* 209 (1969): 1505–10. The diagnostic label "persistent vegetative state" was first coined in 1972. B. Jennett and F. Plum, "Persistent Vegetative State after Brain Damage: A Syndrome in Search of a Name," *Lancet* 1 (1972): 734–37.

11. N. Dubler and D. Nimmons, *Ethics on Call* (New York: Harmony Books, 1992).

12. Hippocratic Corpus, "The Art," in *Ethics in Medicine: Historical Perspectives and Contemporary Concerns,* ed. S. J. Reiser, A. J. Dyck, and W. J. Curran (Cambridge: MIT Press, 1977).

13. D. W. Amundsen, "The Physician's Obligation to Prolong Life: A Medical Duty without Classical Roots," *Hastings Center Report* 8, no. 4 (1978): 23–30.

14. A. A. Lyons and R. J. Petrucelli, *Medicine: An Illustrative History* (New York: Abradele Press, 1987), p. 291.

15. N. S. Jecker, "Knowing When to Stop: The Limits of Medicine," *Hastings Center Report* 21, no. 3 (1991): 6.

16. D. W. Amundsen, personal communication.

17. R. D. Truog, A. S. Brett, and J. Frader, "The Problem with Futility," *New England Journal of Medicine* 326 (1992): 1560–64.

18. J. D. Lantos, P. A. Singer, R. M. Walker, et al., "The Illusion of Futility in Clinical Practice," *American Journal of Medicine* 87 (1989): 81–84.

19. P. Helft, M. Siegler, and J. Lantos, "The Rise and Fall of the Futility Movement." *New England Journal of Medicine* 343 (2000): 293–96.

20. E. D. Pellegrino, "Decisions at the End of Life: The Abuse of the Concept of Futility," *Practical Bioethics* 1 (2005): 3–6.

21. Lantos, Singer, Walker, et al., "The Illusion of Futility in Clinical Practice."

22. M. Angell, "The Case of Helga Wanglie," *New England Journal of Medicine* 325 (1991): 511–12.

23. H. Brody, "The Power to Determine Futility," in *The Healer's Power* (New Haven: Yale University Press, 1992), p. 179.

24. Ibid.

25. J. T. Noonan, "An Almost Absolute Value in History," in *The Morality of Abortion,* ed. J. T. Noonan Jr. (Cambridge: Harvard University Press, 1970), pp. 51–59.

26. P. Singer, *Animal Liberation* (New York: Harper Collins, 2009).

27. N. S. Jecker, "Medical Futility: A Paradigm Analysis," *HEC Forum* 19 (2007): 13–32.

28. D. Hume, *A Treatise of Human Nature,* ed. L. A. Selby-Bigge (New York: Oxford University Press, 1978), p. 73.

29. K. R. Popper, *The Logic of Scientific Discovery* (New York: Basic Books, 1961). With respect to the "idol of certainty," Popper states: "The old scientific ideal of *episteme*—of absolutely certain, demonstrable knowledge—has proved to be an idol. The demand for scientific objectivity makes it inevitable that every scientific statement must remain *tentative for ever.* It may indeed be corroborated, but every corroboration is relative to other statements which, again, are tentative. Only in our subjective experiences of conviction, in our subjective faith, can we be 'absolutely certain.'"

30. L. J. Schneiderman and A. M. Capron, "How Can Hospital Futility Policies Contribute to Establishing Standards of Practice?" *Cambridge Quarterly of Healthcare Ethics* 9 (2000): 524–31.

31. J. D. Lantos, S. H. Miles, M. D. Silverstein, and C. B. Stocking, "Survival after Cardiopulmonary Resuscitation in Babies of Very Low Birthweight: Is CPR Futile?" *New England Journal of Medicine* 318 (1988): 91–95; A. L. Kellermann, D. R. Staves, and B. B. Hackman, "In-Hospital Resuscitation Following Unsuccessful Prehospital Advanced Cardiac Life-Support: 'Heroic Efforts' or an Exercise in Futility?" *Annals of Emergency Medicine* 17 (1988): 589–94; M. J. Bonnin and R. A. Swor, "Outcomes in Unsuccessful Field Resuscitation Attempts," *Annals of Emergency Medicine* 18 (1989): 507–12; D. J. Murphy, A. M. Mur-

ray, B. E. Robinson, and E. W. Campion, "Outcomes of Cardiopulmonary Resuscitation in the Elderly," *Annals of Internal Medicine* 111 (1989): 199–205; K. Faber-Langendoen, "Resuscitation of Patients with Metastatic Cancer: Is Transient Benefit Still Futile?" *Archives of Internal Medicine* 151 (1991): 235–39; W. A. Gray, R. J. Capone, and A. S. Most, "Unsuccessful Emergency Medical Resuscitation: Are Continued Efforts in the Emergency Department Justified?" *New England Journal of Medicine* 325 (1991): 1393–98.

32. C. Sasson, A. L. Kellermann, and B. F. McNally, "Prehospital Termination of Resuscitation in Cases of Refractory Out-of-Hospital Cardiac Arrest," *JAMA* 300 (2008): 1432–38.

33. Plato, *Republic,* bk. 3, trans. E. Hamilton and H. Cairns (Princeton: Princeton University Press, 1980).

34. D. Postema, personal communication.

35. Ibid.

36. A. R. Jonsen, personal communication.

37. D. Rothman, "Strong Medicine: The Ethical Rationing of Health Care," *New York Review of Books* 39 (1992): 33.

38. R. Dworkin, *Life's Dominion* (New York: Vintage Books, 1994), p. 28.

CHAPTER TWO: Why It Is Hard to Say No

1. M. Nussbaum, "Transcending Humanity," in *Love's Knowledge* (New York: Oxford University Press, 1990), p. 365.

2. Ibid.

3. Ibid.

4. D. Callahan, *The Troubled Dream of Life* (New York: Simon and Schuster, 1993), p. 61.

5. H. Brody, "Assisted Death: A Compassionate Response to a Medical Failure," *New England Journal of Medicine* 327 (1992): 1385.

6. K. Lebacz, "Humility in Health Care," *Journal of Medicine and Philosophy* 17 (1992): 291.

7. L. J. Schneiderman, "Exile and PVS," *Hastings Center Report* 20, no. 3 (1990): 5. On minimal or complete unawareness, see note 2 to Chapter 1.

8. J. M. Kriett and M. P Kaye, "The Registry of the International Society for Heart Transplantation: Seventh Official Report, 1990," *Journal of Heart Transplantation* 9 (1990): 323–30; Kriett and Kaye, "Eighth Official Report, 1991," ibid. 10 (1991): 491–98; P. M. Park, "The Transplant Odyssey," *Second Opinion* 12 (1989): 27–32; K. Rolles, "Summary of Clinical Data: Liver Transplantation," in *Organ Transplantation: Current Clinical and Immunological Concepts,* ed. L. Brent and R. A. Sells (London: Balliere Tindall, 1989), pp. 201–5; D. Azoulay, M. M. Linhares, E. Huguet, et al., "Decision for Retransplantation of the Liver: An Experience- and Cost-Based Analysis," *Annals of Surgery* 236 (2002): 713–21; J. F. Markmann, J. S. Markowitz, H. Yersiz, et al., "Long-Term Survival after Retransplantation of the Liver," *Annals of Surgery* 226 (1997): 408–18; J. A. Powelson, A. B. Cosimi, W. D. Lewis, et al., "Hepatic Retransplantation in New England: A Regional Experience and Survival Model," *Transplantation* 55 (1993): 802–6.

9. W. Cather, *Death Comes for the Archbishop* (New York: Alfred A. Knopf, 1951), p. 170.

10. J. Itami, "A Director Boasts of His Scars, and Says He Is Right about Japan's Mob," *New York Times,* August 30, 1992, p. E7.

11. In his novel, *Death with Interruptions* (New York: Harcourt, 2005), the Nobel

Prize–winning José Saramago laments with sly wit "that the undeserved disappearance of so many people in the past could be put down solely to a deplorable weakness of will on the part of previous generations" (p. 6).

12. *The Compact Edition of the Oxford English Dictionary* (New York: Oxford University Press, 1971), s.v. "compassion."

13. F. W. Hafferty, *Into the Valley: Death and the Socialization of Medical Students* (New Haven: Yale University Press, 1991), p. 38.

14. J. Kilner, "Who Shall Be Saved: An African Answer," *Hastings Center Report* 14, no. 3 (1984): 19–22.

15. Epicurus, Letter to Menoeceus.

16. N. S. Jecker and L. J. Schneiderman, "Is Dying Young Worse Than Dying Old?" *Gerontologist* 3 (1994): 66–72.

17. D. M. Studdert, M. M. Mello, W. M. Sage, et al., "Defensive Medicine among High-Risk Specialist Physicians in a Volatile Malpractice Environment," *JAMA* 293 (2005): 2609–17.

18. L. J. Schneiderman and J. E. Fein, "The Limits of Dispute Resolution," *Hastings Center Report* 31, no. 6 (2001): 10–11.

19. G. J. Annas, "Faith (Healing), Hope, and Charity at the FDA: The Politics of AIDS Drug Trials," in *AIDS and the Health Care System,* ed. L. O. Gostin (New Haven: Yale University Press, 1990), p. 194.

20. Nussbaum, "Transcending Humanity," p. 365.

CHAPTER THREE: Why We Must Say No

1. M. Z. Solomon, L. O'Donnell, B. Jennings, et al., "Decisions near the End of Life: Professional Views on Life-Sustaining Treatments," *American Journal of Public Health* 83 (1993): 19.

2. *Barber v. Los Angeles County Superior Court,* 195 Cal. Rptr. 484, 147 Cal. App. 3d 1006 (1983).

3. President's Commission for the Study of Ethical Problems in Medicine and Biomedical and Behavioral Research, *Deciding to Forego Life-Sustaining Treatment* (Washington, DC: U.S. Government Printing Office, 1983), p. 44

4. Solomon et al., "Decisions near the End of Life," p. 19.

5. D. Humphry, *Final Exit* (Eugene, OR: Hemlock Society, 1991).

6. T. M. Pope, "Medical Futility Statutes: No Safe Harbor to Unilaterally Refuse Life Sustaining Medical Treatment," *Tennessee Law Review* 71 (2007): 1–81.

7. Ibid.

8. *Texas Health and Safety Code Annotated,* sec. 166.046.

9. E. D. Pellegrino, "Futility in Medical Decisions: The Word and the Concept," *HEC Forum* 17 (2005): 308–18.

10. T. M. Pope, "Involuntary Passive Euthanasia in U.S. Courts: Reassessing the Judicial Treatment of Medical Futility Cases," *Marquette Elder's Advisor* 9 (2008): 229–63.

11. Pope, "Medical Futility Statutes."

12. Ibid.

13. G. D. Lundberg, "American Health Care System Management Objectives: The Aura of Inevitability Becomes Incarnate," *JAMA* 269 (1993): 2554–55.

14. "Remaking America's Health-Care System," *The Lancet* 374 (2009): 57.

15. P. Farmer and N. Gastineau Campos, "New Malaise: Bioethics and Human Rights in the Global Era," in *Bioethics: An Introduction to the History, Methods, and Practice,* ed. N. S. Jecker, A. R. Jonsen, and R. A. Pearlman, 2nd ed. (Sudbury, MA: Jones and Bartlett, 2007), p. 297.

16. R. Abelson, "Weighing Medical Costs of End-of-Life Care," *New York Times,* December 23, 2009.

17. Council for the American Recovery and Reinvestment Act (ARRA), *Report to the President and the Congress on Comparative Effectiveness Research,* www.hhs.gov/recovery/programs/cer/execsummary.html, accessed December 31, 2009.

18. A. I. Mushlin and H. Ghomrawi, "Health Care Reform and the Need for Comparative-Effectiveness Research," *New England Journal of Medicine* 10 (2010): 1056–58.

19. H. P. Selker and A. J. J. Wool, "Industry Influence on Comparative-Effectiveness Research Funded through Health Care Reform," *New England Journal of Medicine* 361 (2009): 2595–97.

20. The Multi-Society Task Force on PVS, "Medical Aspects of the Persistent Vegetative State, I," *New England Journal of Medicine* 330 (1994): 1499–1508.

21. J. L. Bernat, *Ethical Issues in Neurology,* 3rd ed. (Philadelphia: Lippincott Williams & Wilkins, 2008), p. 295; S. Haidinger and G. Binder, "Prevalence of Persistent Vegetative State/Apallic Syndrome in Vienna," *European Journal of Neurology* 11 (2004): 461–66; J. C. Lavrijsen, J. S. van den Bosch, R. T. Koopmans, and C. van Weel, "Prevalence and Characteristics of Patients in a Vegetative State in Dutch Nursing Homes," *Journal of Neurology, Neurosurgery, and Psychiatry* 76 (2005): 1420–24.

22. D. Callahan, *Setting Limits: Medical Goals in an Aging Society* (New York: Touchstone, 1988), p. 171.

23. R. A. Rettig, "The Policy Debate on Patient Care Financing for Victims of End-Stage Renal Disease," *Law and Contemporary Problems* 40 (1976): 200.

24. G. A. Puckrein and K. Norris, "Medicare End Stage Renal Disease Program: Why We Must Have a Paradigm Shift in Health Care," *National Minority Quality Forum,* December 10, 2007; D. L. Shelton, "Older Transplant Patients, Donors," *Los Angeles Times,* September 20, 2009, p. A4.

25. J. K. Iglehart, "The American Health Care System: The End Stage Renal Disease Program," *New England Journal of Medicine* 328 (1993): 371.

26. U.S. Preventive Services Task Force, "Screening for Breast Cancer: U.S. Preventive Services Task Force Recommendations Statement," *Annals of Internal Medicine* 151 (2009): 716–26; G. Kolata, "Mammogram Debate Took Group Off Guard," *New York Times,* November 20, 2009, p. A22.

27. R. Rosenthal, "One Siamese Twin Survives An Extraordinary Separation," *New York Times,* August 21, 1993; "Twin Who Survived Separation Surgery Dies," *New York Times,* June 10, 1994.

28. R. M. Dworkin, "The Price of Life," *Los Angeles Times,* August 29, 1993, p. M1.

29. A. Taunton-Rigby, Genzyme's senior vice-president of therapeutics, quoted in "New Drug Standard: Economic Value," *New York Times,* January 18, 1993, p. C3.

30. A. Pollack, "A Fortune to Fight Cancer: Cost of Drugs Is Soaring, Defying Reform," *New York Times,* December 5, 2009, p. B1.

31. K. Faber-Langendoen, A. L. Caplan, and P. B. McGlave, "Survival of Adult Bone-

Marrow Transplant Patients Receiving Mechanical Ventilation: A Case for Restricted Use," *Bone Marrow Transplantation* 12 (1993): 501–7.

32. G. D. Rubenfeld and S. W. Crawford, "Withdrawing Life Support from Mechanically Ventilated Recipients of Bone Marrow Transplants: A Case for Evidence-Based Guidelines," *Annals of Internal Medicine* 125 (1996): 625–33.

33. S. C. Schoenbaum, "Toward Fewer Procedures and Better Outcomes," *JAMA* 269 (1993): 794–96.

34. T. S. Kuhn, *The Structure of Scientific Revolutions* (Chicago: University of Chicago Press, 1970).

35. D. Oken, "What to Tell Cancer Patients: A Study of Medical Attitudes," *JAMA* 175 (1961): 1120–28.

36. D. H. Novack, R. Plumer, R. L. Smith, et al., "Changes in Physicians' Attitudes toward Telling the Cancer Patient," *JAMA* 241 (1979): 897–900.

37. The revered physician's advice came from an honored tradition. Oliver Wendell Holmes wrote: "Your patient has no more right to all the truth you know than he has to all the medicine in your saddlebags. . . . He should get only just so much as is good for him. . . . It is a terrible thing to take away hope, every earthly hope, from a fellow creature." In "The Young Practitioner," *Medical Essays*, vol. 9 of *Writings of Oliver Wendell Holmes* (Boston, 1891), p. 388.

38. G. J. Annas, *The Rights of Patients: The Basic ACLU Guide to Patient Rights* (Totowa, NJ: Humana Press, 1992).

39. Rettig, "Patient Care Financing for Victims of End-Stage Renal Disease."

40. N. S. Jecker, "The Role of Intimate Others in Medical Decision-Making," *Gerontologist* 30 (1990): 65–71; H. H. Hiatt, "Protecting the Medical Commons: Who Is Responsible?" *New England Journal of Medicine* 293 (1975): 235–41; G. Hardin, "The Tragedy of the Commons," *Science* 162 (1968): 1243–48; J. Hardwig, "What about the Family?" *Hastings Center Report* 20, no. 2 (1990): 5–10; N. S. Jecker, "Being a Burden on Others," *Journal of Clinical Ethics* 4 (1993): 16–20.

41. L. J. Schneiderman and R. M. Kaplan, "Fear of Dying and HIV Infection vs. Hepatitis B Infection," *American Journal of Public Health* 82 (1992): 584–86.

42. W. Cather, *Death Comes for the Archbishop* (New York: Vintage Books, 1990), p. 16.

CHAPTER FOUR: Families Who Say, "Do Everything!"

1. N. S. Weiss, J. M. Liff, C. L. Ure, J. H. Ballard, G. H. Abbott, and J. R. Daling, "Mortality in Women Following Hip Fracture," *Journal of Chronic Disease* 36 (1983): 879–82; C. W. Miller, "Survival and Ambulation Following Hip Fracture," *Journal of Bone and Joint Surgery* 60-A (1978): 930–34; B. L. White, W. D. Fisher, and C. A. Laurin, "Rate of Mortality for Elderly Patients after Fracture of the Hip in the 1980s," ibid. 69–A (1987): 1335–39; S. R. Cummings, D. M. Black, and S. M. Rubin, "Lifetime Risks of Hip, Colles', or Vertebral Fracture and Coronary Heart Disease among White Postmenopausal Women," *Archives of Internal Medicine* 149 (1989): 2445–48.

2. S. H. Miles, "Informed Demand for 'Non-beneficial' Medical Treatment," *New England Journal of Medicine* 325 (1991): 512–15.

3. Ibid.

4. Ibid.

5. R. E. Cranford, "Helga Wanglie's Ventilator," *Hastings Center Report* 21, no. 4 (1991): 23–24.

6. Miles, "Informed Demand for 'Non-beneficial' Medical Treatment."

7. M. A. Rie, "The Limits of a Wish," *Hastings Center Report* 21, no. 4 (1991): 24–25.

8. E. H. Cassem, personal communication. See also T. A. Brennan, "Ethics Committees and Decisions to Limit Care," *JAMA* 260 (1988): 803–7.

9. A. Goodnough, "Court Voids Law Keeping Woman Alive," *New York Times,* September 24, 2004, p. A1.

10. Ibid.

11. C. Baranauckas, "Florida Judge Overturns Law in Right-to-Die Case," *New York Times,* May 6, 2004.

12. Pope John Paul II, "Address of John Paul II to the Participants in the 'International Congress on Life-Sustaining Treatments and Vegetative State: Scientific Advances and Ethical Dilemmas,'" March 20, 2004. In point 4 of this speech, the pope said that "the administration of water and food, even when provided by artificial means, always represents a natural means of preserving life, not a medical act." See also Congregation for the Doctrine of the Faith, "Responses to Certain Questions of the United States Conference of Catholic Bishops Concerning Artificial Nutrition and Hydration," August 1, 2007, and "The Revision of Directive 58 of Ethical and Religious Directives for Catholic Health Care Services," December 16, 2009. All are available through the National Catholic Bioethics Center (NCBC), www.ncbcenter.org.

13. O. C. Snead, "The (Surprising) Truth about *Schiavo*: A Defeat for the Cause of Autonomy," *Constitutional Commentary* 22 (2005): 383–404.

14. N. Daniels, *Am I My Parents' Keeper?* (New York: Oxford University Press, 1988), p. viii.

15. J. J. Paris and F. E. Reardon, "Physician Refusal of Requests for Futile or Ineffective Interventions," *Cambridge Quarterly of Health Care Ethics* 2 (1992): 127.

16. M. Angell, "The Case of Helga Wanglie: A New Kind of 'Right to Die' Case," *New England Journal of Medicine* 325 (1991): 511–12. See also A. M. Capron, "In re Helga Wanglie," *Hastings Center Report* 21, no. 5 (1991): 26–28; F. Ackerman, "The Significance of a Wish," ibid. 21, no. 4 (1991): 27–29; S. M. Wolf, "Conflict between Doctor and Patient," *Law, Medicine, and Health Care* 16, nos. 3–4 (1988): 197–203; T. A. Brennan, "Silent Decisions: Limits of Consent and the Terminally Ill Patient," ibid., pp. 204–9.

17. Paris and Reardon, "Physician Refusal of Requests," p. 128.

18. A. S. Brett and L. B. McCullough, "When Patients Request Specific Interventions," *New England Journal of Medicine* 315 (1986): 1349.

19. E. Pellegrino, "Ethics in AIDS Treatment Decisions," *Origins* 19 (1990): 539–44; D. W. Brock and S. A. Wartman, "When Competent Patients Make Irrational Choices," *New England Journal of Medicine* 322 (1990): 1595–99.

20. J. R. Zuckerman, letter to editor, *New York Times,* August 22, 1992.

21. R. M. Veatch and C. M. Spicer, "Medically Futile Care: The Role of the Physician in Setting Limits," *American Journal of Law and Medicine* 18, nos. 1–2 (1992): 17.

22. L. J. Schneiderman, K. Faber-Langendoen, and N. S. Jecker, "Beyond Futility to an Ethic of Care," *American Journal of Medicine* 96 (1994): 110–14.

23. U.S. Department of Health and Human Services, Agency for Health Care Policy and Research, Clinical Practice Guideline, *Acute Pain Management: Operative or Medical Procedures and Trauma* (Rockville, MD: Agency for Health Care Policy and Research,

1992); S. Hauerwas, "Care," in *Encyclopedia of Bioethics,* ed. W. T. Reich (New York: Free Press, 1978), 1:145–50; A. R. Nelson, "Humanism and the Art of Medicine: Our Commitment to Care," *JAMA* 262 (1989): 1228–30.

24. N. S. Jecker and W. T. Reich, "Contemporary Ethics of Care," in *Encyclopedia of Bioethics,* 3rd ed., ed. S. G. Post (New York: Macmillan Reference USA, 2004), p. 367.

25. N. S. Jecker and J. D. Self, "Separating Care and Cure: An Analysis of Historical and Contemporary Images of Nursing and Medicine," *Journal of Medicine and Philosophy* 16 (1991): 285–306; S. A. Gadow, "Nurse and Patient: The Caring Relationship," in *Caring, Curing, Coping: Nurse, Physician, Patient Relationships,* ed. A. Bishop and J. Scudder (Birmingham: University of Alabama Press, 1985), pp. 31–43.

26. N. S. Jecker, "Justice and the Private Sphere," *Public Affairs Quarterly* 8 (1994): 255–66; L. Blum, "Care," in *The Encyclopedia of Ethics,* ed. L. C. Becker and C. B. Becker (New York: Garland Publishing, 1992), 1:125.

27. Jecker and Self, "Separating Care and Cure."

28. Ibid., p. 292.

29. Ibid., p. 295.

30. N. Coyle, "Continuity of Care for the Cancer Patient with Chronic Pain," *Cancer* 63 (1989): 2289–93; T. D. Walsh, "Continuing Care in a Medical Center: The Cleveland Clinic Foundation Palliative Care Service," *Journal of Pain and Symptom Management* 5, no. 5 (1990): 273–78.

31. L. A. Printz, "Terminal Dehydration: A Compassionate Treatment," *Archives of Internal Medicine* 152 (1992): 697–700; P. Schmitz and M. O'Brien, "Observations on Nutrition and Hydration in Dying Cancer Patients," in *By No Extraordinary Means,* ed. J. Lynn (Bloomington: Indiana University Press, 1986), pp. 29–38.

32. R. J. Sullivan, "Accepting Death without Artificial Nutrition or Hydration," *Journal of General Internal Medicine* 8 (1993): 220–24.

33. T. E. Quill, "Doctor, I Want to Die; Will You Help Me?" *JAMA* 270 (1993): 871.

34. S. Manning and L. J. Schneiderman, "Miracles or Limits: What Message from the Medical Market Place?" *HEC Forum* 8, no. 2 (1996): 103–8.

35. K. Faber-Langendoen, "Medical Futility: Values, Goals, and Certainty," *Journal of Laboratory and Clinical Medicine* 120 (1992): 831–35.

36. Veatch and Spicer, "Medically Futile Care."

37. L. J. Schneiderman, T. Gilmer, H. D. Teetzel, et al., "Effect of Ethics Consultations on Nonbeneficial Life-Sustaining Treatments in the Intensive Care Setting: A Randomized Controlled Trial," *JAMA* 290, no. 9 (2004): 1166–72.

38. L. J. Schneiderman, *Embracing Our Mortality: Hard Choices in an Age of Medical Miracles* (New York: Oxford University Press, 2008).

39. M. Webb, *The Good Death: The New American Search to Reshape the End of Life* (New York: Bantam, 1997).

CHAPTER FIVE: Futility and Rationing

1. "Remaking America's Health-Care System," *The Lancet* 374 (2009): 57.

2. E. Ginzberg, "A Hard Look at Cost Containment," *New England Journal of Medicine* 316 (1987): 1151–54.

3. T. Gilmer, L. J. Schneiderman, H. Teetzel, et al., "The Costs of Nonbeneficial Treatment in the Intensive Care Setting," *Health Affairs* 24 (2005): 961–71.

4. M. McGregor, "Technology and the Allocation of Resources," *New England Journal of Medicine* 320 (1989): 118–20.

5. L. J. Blackhall, "Must We Always Use CPR?" *New England Journal of Medicine* 17 (1987): 1281–84.

6. T. Tomlinson and H. Brody, "Ethics and Communication in Do-Not-Resuscitate Orders," *New England Journal of Medicine* 318 (1988): 43–46.

7. J. Risen, "Expert Panel Brews Bitter Tonic for U.S. Fiscal Malaise," *Los Angeles Times*, August 30, 1992, p. A10.

8. D. Callahan, *Setting Limits: Medical Goals in an Aging Society* (New York: Simon and Schuster, 1987).

9. We draw on a number of studies in making these claims, including D. J. Murphy, A. M. Murray, B. E. Robinson, et al., "Outcomes of Cardiopulmonary Resuscitation in the Elderly," *Annals of Internal Medicine* 111 (1989): 199–205; B. J. Gersh, R. A. Kronmal, R. L. Frye, et al., "Coronary Arteriography and Coronary Artery Bypass Surgery: Morbidity and Mortality in Patients Ages 65 Years and Older," *Circulation* 67 (1983): 483–91; T. Randall, "Successful Liver Transplantation in Older Patients Raises New Hopes, Challenges, Ethics Questions," *JAMA* 264 (1990): 428–30; J. D. Pirsch, R. J. Stratta, M. J. Armbrust, et al., "Cadaveric Renal Transplantation with Cyclosporine in Patients More Than 60 Years of Age," *Transplantation* 47 (1989): 259–61; M. P. Hosking, M. A. Warner, C. M. Lobdell, et al., "Outcomes of Surgery in Patients 90 Years of Age or Older," *JAMA* 261 (1989): 1909–15; C. B. Begg, J. L. Cohen, J. Ellerton, "Are the Elderly Predisposed to Toxicity from Cancer Chemotherapy?" *Cancer Clinical Trials* 3 (1980): 369–74; L. Westlie, A. Umen, S. Nestrud, et al., "Mortality, Morbidity, and Life Satisfaction in the Very Old Dialysis Patient," *Transactions of the American Society of Artificial Internal Organs* 30 (1984): 21–30.

10. N. Daniels, *Am I My Parents' Keeper?* (New York: Oxford University Press, 1988).

11. R. M. Veatch, *A Theory of Medical Ethics* (New York: Basic Books, 1981).

12. A. S. Brett and L. B. McCullough, "When Patients Request Specific Interventions," *New England Journal of Medicine* 315 (1986): 1347–51.

13. J. Hammond and C. G. Ward, "Decisions Not to Treat: 'Do-Not-Resuscitate' Order for the Burn Patient in the Acute Setting," *Critical Care Medicine* 17 (1989): 136–38; J. D. Lantos, S. H. Miles, M. D. Silverstein, and C. B. Stocking, "Survival after Cardiopulmonary Resuscitation in Babies of Very Low Birthweight: Is CPR Futile Therapy?" *New England Journal of Medicine* 318 (1988): 91–95; G. E. Taffet, T. A. Teasdale, and R. J. Luchi, "In-Hospital Cardiopulmonary Resuscitation," *JAMA* 260 (1988): 2069–72; D. J. Murphy, "Do-Not-Resuscitate Orders: Time for Reappraisal in Long-Term Care Institutions," *JAMA* 260 (1988): 2098–2101; L. J. Schneiderman and R. G. Spragg, "Ethical Decisions in Discontinuing Mechanical Ventilation," *New England Journal of Medicine* 318 (1988): 984–88; J. J. Paris, R. K. Crone, and F. Reardon, "Physicians' Refusal of Requested Treatment: The Case of Baby L," *New England Journal of Medicine* 322 (1990): 1012–15; D. V. Schapira, J. Studnicki, D. D. Bradham, et al., "Intensive Care, Survival, and Expense of Treating Critically Ill Cancer Patients," *JAMA* 269 (1993): 783–86.

14. President's Commission for the Study of Ethical Problems in Medicine and Biomedical and Behavioral Research, *Securing Access to Health Care*, vol. 1 (Washington, DC: Government Printing Office, 1983), pp. 46–47.

15. C. Gilligan and S. Pollak, "The Vulnerable and the Invulnerable Physician," in *Mapping the Moral Domain*, ed. C. Gilligan, J. V. Ward, and J. M. Taylor (Cambridge: Harvard University Press, 1988), pp. 245–62.

16. Ibid.
17. N. Daniels, "Why Saying No to Patients in the United States Is So Hard," *New England Journal of Medicine* 314 (1986): 1380–83.

CHAPTER SIX: Medical Futility in a Litigious Society

1. R. F. Weir and L. O. Gostin, "Decisions to Abate Life-Sustaining Treatment for Nonautonomous Patients," *JAMA* 264 (1990): 1846–53.
2. L. J. Nelson and R. E. Cranford, "Legal Advice, Moral Paralysis, and the Death of Samuel Linares," *Law, Medicine, and Health Care* 17 (1989): 316–24.
3. "America's Parasite Economy," *Economist*, October 10, 1992, p. 21.
4. J. H. Birnbaum, "The Road to Riches Is Called K Street," *Washington Post*, June 22, 2005.
5. Quoted in D. D. Kirkpatrick, "Intended to Rein In Lobbyists, Law Sends Them Underground," *New York Times*, January 18, 2010, p. A1.
6. D. M. Studdert, M. M. Mello, W. M. Sage, et al., "Defensive Medicine among High-Risk Specialist Physicians in a Volatile Malpractice Environment," *JAMA* 293 (2005): 2609–17.
7. B. McCormick, "Study: Defensive Medicine Costs Nearly $10,000,000,000," *American Medical News*, February 15, 1993, p. 4.
8. D. MacCourt and J. Bernstein, "Medical Error Reduction and Tort Reform through Private, Contractually Based Quality Medicine Societies," *American Journal of Law & Medicine* 35 (2009): 505–61.
9. D. Leonhardt, "Medical Malpractice System Breeds More Waste," *New York Times*, September 23, 2009.
10. A. M. Vintzileos, D. J. Nochimson, E. R. Guzman, R. A. Knuppel, M. Lake, and S. Schifrin, "Intrapartum Electronic Fetal Heart Rate Monitoring versus Intermittent Auscultation: A Meta-Analysis," *Obstetrics & Gynecology* 85 (1995): 149–55; American College of Obstetricians and Gynecologists, ACOG Practice Bulletin No. 75, "Intrapartum Fetal Heart Rate Monitoring," *Obstetrics & Gynecology* 106 (2005): 1453–61; S. B. Thacker, D. Stroup, and M. Chang, "Continuous Electronic Heart Rate Monitoring for Fetal Assessment during Labor," *Cochrane Database of Systematic Reviews* 2 (2001): CD000063.
11. Committee to Study Medical Professional Liability and the Delivery of Obstetrical Care, Division of Health Promotion and Disease Prevention, Institute of Medicine, *Medical Professional Liability and the Delivery of Obstetrical Care* 1 (1989): 81.
12. P. W. Huber, *Galileo's Revenge: Junk Science in the Courtroom* (New York: Basic Books, 1993), p. 87.
13. J. H. Ferguson, M. Dubinsky, and P. J. Kirsch, "Court-Ordered Reimbursement for Unproven Medical Technology," *JAMA* 269 (1993): 2116–21.
14. *Daubert v. Merrell Dow Pharmaceuticals*, 113 S. Ct. 2786 (1993); G. J. Annas, "Scientific Evidence in the Courtroom: The Death of the Frye Rule," *New England Journal of Medicine* 330 (1994): 1018–21; J. E. Bertin and M. S. Henifin, "Science, Law, and the Search for Truth in the Courtroom: Lesson from *Daubert v. Merrell Dow*," *Journal of Law, Medicine, and Ethics* 22 (1994): 6–20.
15. *General Electric v. Joiner*, 522 U.S. 136 (1997); *Moore v. Ashland Chemical*, 151 F.3d 269 (1998); *Canavan v. Brigham and Women's Hospital*, 48 Mass. App. Ct. 297 (1999).
16. A. R. Localio, A. G. Lothers, J, M. Bengtson, et al., "Relationship between Malpractice Claims and Caesarean Delivery," *JAMA* 269 (1993): 366–73.

17. Huber, *Galileo's Revenge*, 179.

18. L. Esserman, Y. Shieh, and I. Thompson, "Rethinking Screening for Breast Cancer and Prostate Cancer," *JAMA* 302 (2009): 1685–92.

19. G. Kolata, "Patients' Lawyers Lead Insurers to Pay for Unproven Treatments," *New York Times*, March 28, 1994, p. A1; G. Harris, "Where Cancer Progress Is Rare, One Man Says No," *New York Times*, September 16, 2009, p. A28.

20. H. Meyer, "Breast Study Woes Preview Reform Barriers," *American Medical News*, March 8, 1993, p. 1.

21. Kolata, "Patients' Lawyers Lead Insurers to Pay for Unproven Treatments"; Harris, "Where Cancer Progress Is Rare, One Man Says No."

22. E. A. Stadtmauer, A. O'Neill, L. J. Goldstein, et al., "Conventional-Dose Chemotherapy Compared with High-Dose Chemotherapy plus Autologous Hematopoietic Stem-Cell Transplantation for Metastatic Breast Cancer," *New England Journal of Medicine* 342 (2000): 1069–76; C. Farquhar, J. Marjoribanks, R. Basser, S. Hetrick, and A. Lethaby, "High Dose Chemotherapy and Autologous Bone Marrow or Stem Cell Transplantation versus Conventional Chemotherapy for Women with Metastatic Breast Cancer," *Cochrane Database of Systematic Reviews* 3 (2005): CD003142.

23. L. K. Stell, "Stopping Treatment on Grounds of Futility: A Role for Institutional Policy," *St. Louis University Public Law Review* 11 (1992): 489.

24. *In re Quinlan*, 70 N.J. 10, 355 A.2d 647 (1976).

25. A. Meisel, "Legal Myths about Terminating Life Support," *Archives of Internal Medicine* 151 (1991): 1498–1502.

26. M. B. Kapp, "'Cookbook' Medicine: A Legal Perspective," *Archives of Internal Medicine* 150 (1990): 497.

27. Nelson and Cranford, "Legal Advice," p. 321.

28. S. V. McCrary, J. W. Swanson, H. S. Perkins, and W. J. Winslade, "Treatment Decisions for Terminally Ill Patients: Physicians' Legal Defensiveness and Knowledge of Medical Law," *Law, Medicine, and Health Care* 20 (1992): 364–76.

29. *Barber v. Los Angeles County Superior Court*, 195 Cal. Rptr. 484, 147 Cal. App. 3d 1006 (1983).

30. P. Schmitz and M. O'Brien, "Observations on Nutrition and Hydration in Dying Cancer Patients," in *By No Extraordinary Means*, ed. J. Lynn (Bloomington: Indiana University Press, 1986), pp. 29–38.

31. I. Byock and L. Cohen, personal communication, 2009.

32. *In re Jobes*, 529 A.2d 434 (NJ 1987).

33. A. Meisel, "The Role of Litigation in End of Life Care: A Reappraisal," in *Improving End of Life Care: Why Has It Been So Difficult?* Hastings Center Report Special Report 35, no. 6 (2005): S47–51.

34. Meisel, "Legal Myths about Terminating Life Support."

35. L. J. Schneiderman, R. A. Pearlman, R. M. Kaplan, et al., "Relationship of General Advance Directive Instructions to Specific Life-Sustaining Treatment Preferences in Patients with Serious Illness," *Archives of Internal Medicine* 152 (1992): 2114–22.

36. *Conservatorship of Wendland*, 26 Cal. 4th 519 (2001), no. S087265.

37. L. J. Schneiderman, *Embracing Our Mortality: Hard Choices in an Age of Medical Miracles* (New York: Oxford University Press, 2008), pp. 32–42.

38. Several states have statutes (modeled after a California advance directive provision, since rescinded) that allow persons completing a "directive to physicians" to re-

quest that every possible treatment be employed in the event they become incompetent, whether or not a treatment is beneficial or futile. Thus, a patient in Nevada can direct: "I desire that my life be prolonged to the greatest extent possible, without regard to my condition, the chances I have for recovery or long-term survival, or the costs of the procedures" (Durable Power of Attorney for Health Care, Nev. Rev. Sta. Ann 449, 800 [1993]). The practical effect of these statutes remains to be seen. However, they may discourage health providers in these states who seek to practice responsible medicine (including providing comfort care) rather than pursuing futile life-prolongation in dying patients.

Also as we note in this chapter, the Terri Schiavo case spurred a disturbing new tactic: A coalition of "right-to-life" activists, including conservative Catholics and politicians, evangelicals, and splinter groups from disability rights organizations are directing their efforts in the courts and state legislatures seeking laws that prohibit withdrawal of tube feedings under any circumstance, permit pharmacists to refrain from providing birth control medications, and invalidate advance directives, such as living wills. We have already described in Chapter 4 the issues brought to court in the case of Helga Wanglie, in which the family, claiming that a miracle might occur, demanded aggressive life support of an irrevocably unconscious woman. And as noted already in Chapter 5, the most notorious example of the court being called on to force medicine to seek a miracle is *In the Matter of Baby K*.

Baby K was born in October 1992 at Fairfax Hospital in Falls Church, Virginia, with a condition known as anencephaly, a congenital absence of most of the brain. The vast majority of infants with anencephaly die within a few days; none ever develops anything remotely resembling consciousness. Rather than allow the infant to die peacefully, however, the physicians put her on a ventilator, even though they considered the treatment medically futile. The mother disagreed, and insisted that all life-prolonging treatments be continued. The child was moved to a nursing home, but was brought back to the hospital several times for treatment when she manifested breathing difficulties. After the child had survived some 17 months, the hospital finally went to court for permission to refuse to aggressively treat the child if she returned again, arguing that the very nature of anencephaly rendered such treatment futile. The hospital lost in district court and again in the U.S. Court of Appeals by a 2 to 1 vote. The appeals court panel invoked the Emergency Medical Treatment and Active Labor Act, an antidumping law intended to protect seriously ill patients from being dangerously kicked out of emergency facilities because of financial considerations—a move that in this case was inappropriate, because all the child's hospital bills are being paid for by Kaiser Permanente, the mother's insurer.

The lower court also cited what lawyer Marshall Kapp calls a legal "wild card," the Americans with Disabilities Act (ADA). Under this civil rights legislation, health care providers, like other public and private entities, are forbidden to discriminate in the services they provide solely on the basis of a recipient's disability and are required to make "reasonable accommodations" for the sake of disabled recipients. But, as Kapp points out, "If a particular medical intervention truly is futile, no accommodation the provider might make would qualify the patient to benefit from that intervention, and the ADA should be irrelevant. Nonetheless, little guidance exists yet for interpreting the many, often intentional, ambiguities contained in this new law. It remains to be seen whether patients or surrogates will be able to invoke the ADA, by threat or litigation, to frustrate provider wishes to abate futile care on the grounds of discrimination against the disabled." M. B. Kapp, "Futile Medical Treatment: A Review of the Ethical Arguments and Legal Holdings," *Journal of General Internal Medicine* 9 (1994): 170–77. For another excellent discussion of the legal aspects of medical futility, see F. H. Marsh and A. Staver, "Physician Authority for Unilateral DNR Orders," *Journal of Legal Medicine* 12 (1993): 115–65.

CHAPTER SEVEN: Ethical Implications of Medical Futility

1. *Superintendent of Belcherton State School v. Saikewicz,* 370 N.E. 2d. 417 (1977); *Patricia E. Brophy vs. New England Sinai Hospital, Inc.,* N-4152 S.J.C. (1985); *Cruzan v. Director, Missouri Department of Health,* 497 U.S. 261 (1990).

2. G. Kolata, "Court Ruling Limits Rights of Patients: Care Deemed Futile May Be Withheld," *New York Times,* April 22, 1995, p. 6; J. J. Paris, E. H. Cassem, G. W. Dec, and F. E. Reardon, "Use of a DNR Order over Family Objections: The Case of *Gilgunn v. MCH," Journal of Intensive Care Medicine* 14 (1999): 41–45.

3. C. Sasson, A. L. Kellermann, and B. F. McNally, "Prehospital Termination of Resuscitation in Cases of Refractory Out-of-Hospital Cardiac Arrest," *JAMA* 300 (2008): 1432–38.

4. K. Faber-Langendoen, "Resuscitation of Patients with Metastatic Cancer: Is Transient Benefit Still Futile?" *Archives of Internal Medicine* 151 (1991): 235–39.

5. President's Commission for the Study of Ethical Problems in Medicine and Biomedical and Behavioral Research, *Deciding to Forego Life-Sustaining Treatment* (Washington, DC: Government Printing Office, 1983), p. 44; American Thoracic Society, Bioethics Task Force, "Withholding and Withdrawing Life-Sustaining Therapy," *Annals of Internal Medicine* 115 (1991): 478–85; Task Force on Ethics of the Society of Critical Care Medicine, "Consensus Report on the Ethics of Forgoing Life-Sustaining Treatments in the Critically Ill," *Critical Care Medicine* 18 (1990): 1436.

6. H. T. Engelhardt Jr., *The Foundations of Bioethics,* 2nd ed. (New York: Oxford University Press, 1996).

7. R. Veatch, "The Impossibility of a Morality Internal to Medicine," *Journal of Medicine and Philosophy* 26 (2001): 621–42.

8. N. S. Jecker, "Health Care Reform: What History Doesn't Teach," *Theoretical Medicine and Bioethics* 26 (2005): 277–305.

9. Hippocratic Oath, in *Ethics in Medicine: Historical Perspective and Contemporary Concerns,* ed. J. S. Reiser, A. J. Dyck, and W. J. Curran (Cambridge: MIT Press, 1977), p. 5.

10. Plato, *Gorgias,* in *Plato: The Collected Dialogues,* ed. E. Hamilton and H. Cairns (Princeton: Princeton University Press, 1964), p. 262.

11. Plato, *Charmides,* in Hamilton and Cairns, ed., *Plato,* p. 103.

12. E. Pellegrino, "The Goals and Ends of Medicine: How Are They to Be Defined?" in *The Goals of Medicine: The Forgotten Issue in Health Care Reform,* ed. M. Hanson and D. Callahan (Washington, DC: Georgetown University Press, 1999), pp. 55–68. See also E. Pellegrino and D. C. Thomasma, *For the Patient's Good: The Restoration of Beneficence in Health Care* (New York: Oxford University Press, 1988).

13. H. Brody and F. G. Miller, "The Internal Morality of Medicine," *Journal of Medicine and Philosophy* 23 (1998): 386–87.

14. C. Holzer and M. Holzer, "Brain Function after Resuscitation from Cardiac Arrest," *Current Opinion in Critical Care* 10 (2004): 213–17; R. G. Geocadin and S. M. Eleff,

"Cardiac Arrest Resuscitation: Neurologic Prognostication and Brain Death," *Current Opinion in Critical Care* 14 (2008): 261–68.

15. C. van Walraven, A. J. Forster, and I. G. Stiell, "Derivation of a Clinical Decision Rule for the Discontinuation of In-Hospital Cardiac Arrest Resuscitations," *Archives of Internal Medicine* 159 (1999): 129–34; C. van Walraven, A. J. Forster, D. C. Parish, et al., "Validation of a Clinical Decision Aid to Discontinue In-Hospital Cardiac Arrest Resuscitations," *JAMA* 285 (2001): 1602–6; M. A. Peberdy, J. P. Ornato, G. L. Larkin, et al., "Survival from In-Hospital Cardiac Arrest during Nights and Weekends," *JAMA* 299 (2008): 785–92; P. S. Chan, G. Nichol, H. M. Krumholz, et al., "Racial Differences in Survival after In-Hospital Cardiac Arrest," *JAMA* 302 (2009): 1195–1201; G. B. Young, "Clinical Practice. Neurologic Prognosis after Cardiac Arrest," *New England Journal of Medicine* 361 (2009): 605–11; N. K. Choudry, S. Choudry, and P. A. Singer, "CPR for Patients Labeled DNR: The Role of the Limited Aggressive Therapy Order," *Annals of Internal Medicine* 138 (2003): 654–68; S. A. Bernard, T. W. Gray, M. D. Buist, et al., "Treatment of Comatose Survivors of Out-of-Hospital Cardiac Arrest with Induced Hypothermia," *New England Journal of Medicine* 346 (2002): 557–63.

16. President's Commission, *Deciding to Forego,* p. 44.

17. D. Humphrey, *Final Exit* (Eugene, OR: Hemlock Society, 1991).

18. President's Commission, *Deciding to Forego,* p. 44.

19. Hastings Center, *Guidelines on the Termination of Life-Sustaining Treatment and the Care of the Dying* (Indianapolis: Indiana University Press, 1987), p. 19.

20. American Medical Association, Council on Ethical and Judicial Affairs, "Guidelines for the Appropriate Use of Do-Not-Resuscitate Orders," *JAMA* 265 (1991): 1870; American Thoracic Society, "Life-Sustaining Therapy," p. 481; Task Force on Ethics, "Consensus Report"; Society of Critical Care Medicine Ethics Committee, "Consensus Statement on the Triage of Critically Ill Patients" (1993), *JAMA* 271 (1994): 1200–1203; AMA-YPS Handbook Review: HOD Reference Committee on Amendments to Constitution and Bylaws, www.ama-assn.org/ama1/pub/upload/mm/17/gridcandb.pdf.

21. L. J. Schneiderman, N. S. Jecker, and A. R. Jonsen, "Medical Futility: Response to Critiques," *Annals of Internal Medicine* 125 (1996): 669–74.

22. T. E. Finucane, "Life-Prolonging Treatments Late in Life," *Journal of General Internal Medicine* 8 (1993): 399–400.

23. H. K. Beecher, "The Powerful Placebo," *JAMA* 159 (1955): 1602–6; H. Brody and A. Yates, "The Placebo Response," in *Behavior and Medicine,* ed. D. Wedding (St. Louis: Mosby Yearbook, 1990).

24. J. Katz, *The Silent World of Doctor and Patient* (New York: Free Press, 1984).

25. L. J. Schneiderman and J. E. Fein, "The Limits of Dispute Resolution," *Hastings Center Report* 31, no. 6 (2001): 10–11.

26. M. Battin, "Voluntary Euthanasia and the Risk of Abuse: Can We Learn Anything from the Netherlands?" *Law, Medicine, and Health Care* 20 (1992): 137.

27. Ibid.

28. J. W. Walters, *What Is a Person? An Ethical Exploration* (Urbana: University of Illinois Press, 1997).

29. J. T. Noonan Jr., "Development in Moral Doctrine," *Theological Studies* 54 (1993): 669.

30. C. Curran, *Catholic Moral Theology in Dialogue* (Notre Dame: Fides Publishers, 1972), p. 168.

31. McBrien on the *McNeil/Lehrer News Hour*, August 12, 1993.

32. J. Reitman, personal communication.

33. Ibid.

34. B. F. Herring, *Jewish Ethics and Halakah for Our Time* (New York: Yeshiva University Press, 1984), p. 71. For original Halakhah sources see also Yoma 85a: *Mishnah*: If a person is found alive under a fallen house [on the Sabbath] the debris may be removed. *Gemara*: Isn't this obvious? The answer is that this teaches us that this may be done even if only to permit him to live for a short while. *Meiri*: If, when they remove the debris, they examine his breath and find him still alive, they can complete the removal even though he cannot live more than an hour; for in that hour he may repent and utter the confession.

35. I. Jakobovitz, "The Dying and Their Treatment in Jewish Law: Preparation for Death and Euthanasia, *Hebrew Medical Journal* 2 (1961): 251.

36. F. Rosner, J. D. Bleich, and M. M. Brayer, *Jewish Bioethics* (New York: Hebrew Publishing, 1979), pp. 263, 264.

37. A. Steinberg, "A Jewish Perspective on the Four Principles," in *Principles of Health Care Ethics*, ed. R. Gillon (New York: John Wiley, 1994).

38. Noonan, "Moral Doctrine," p. 677.

39. Herring, *Jewish Ethics*, p. 71; Steinberg, "A Jewish Perspective."

40. J. Warren, *Facing Death: Epicurus and His Critics* (Oxford: Oxford University Press, 2004).

CHAPTER EIGHT: The Way It Is Now: For Patients

1. *In the Matter of Westchester County Medical Center, on Behalf of Mary O'Connor*, 72 N.Y. 2d 517, 531 N.E. 2d 607, 534 N.Y.S. 2d 886 (1988).

2. L. Ganzini, E. R. Goy, L. L. Miller, et al., "Nurses' Experiences with Hospice Patients Who Refuse Food and Fluids to Hasten Death," *New England Journal of Medicine* 349 (2003): 359–65; L. A. Printz, "Terminal Dehydration: A Compassionate Treatment," *Archives of Internal Medicine* 152 (1992): 697–700; S. H. Wanzer, D. D. Federman, S. J. Adelstein, et al., "The Physician's Responsibility toward Hopelessly Ill Patients: A Second Look," *New England Journal of Medicine* 320 (1989): 844–49; L. J. Schneiderman and R. G. Spragg, "Ethical Decisions in Discontinuing Mechanical Ventilation," *New England Journal of Medicine* 318 (1988): 984–88; M. Angell, "The Quality of Mercy," *New England Journal of Medicine* 306 (1982): 98–99; R. J. Sullivan, "Accepting Death without Artificial Nutrition or Hydration," *Journal of General Internal Medicine* 8 (1993): 220–24; R. M. McCann, W. J. Hall, and A. Groth-Juncker, "Comfort Care for Terminally Ill Patients: The Appropriate Use of Nutrition and Hydration," *JAMA* 272 (1994): 1263–66; J. D. McCue, "The Naturalness of Dying," *JAMA* 273 (1995): 1039–43.

3. *In re O'Conner*, 72 N.Y. 2d at 533, 531 N.E. 2d at 615, 534 N.Y.S. 2d at 894.

4. Ibid., 72 N.Y. 2d at 544, 531 N.E. 2d at 622, 534 N.Y.S. 2d at 901.

5. R. M. Dworkin, *Life's Dominion* (New York: Alfred A. Knopf, 1993).

6. R. J. Blendon, U. S. Szalay, and R. A. Knox, "Should Physicians Aid Their Patients in Dying?" *JAMA* 267 (1992): 2658–62; M. DiCamillo and M. Field, "Continued Support for Doctor-Assisted Suicide: Most Would Want Their Physician to Assist Them If They Were Incurably Ill and Wanted to Die," The Field Poll, Release 2188, Field Research Corporation, March 15, 2006.

7. *In re O'Connor,* 72 N.Y. 2d at 551, 531 N.E. 2d at 626, 534 N.Y.S. 2d at 905.

8. D. Callahan, "Medical Futility, Medical Necessity: The Problem-without-a-Name," *Hastings Center Report* 21, no. 4 (1991): 34.

9. D. Yankelovich, *Coming to Public Judgment: Making Democracy Work in a Complex World* (Syracuse, NY: Syracuse University Press, 1991), p. 5.

10. L. Saad, "Public Opinion about Abortion: An In-Depth Review," at www.gallup .com/poll/9904/public-opinion-about-abortion-indepth-review.aspx, accessed October 12, 2009.

11. Yankelovich, *Coming to Public Judgment,* pp. 5, 28.

12. B. Jennings, "Possibilities of Consensus: Toward Democratic Moral Discourse," *Journal of Medicine and Philosophy* 16 (1991): 462.

13. Yankelovich, *Coming to Public Judgment,* p. 75.

14. Ibid., p. 65.

15. D. M. Mirvis, "Physicians' Autonomy: The Relation between Public and Professional Expectations," *New England Journal of Medicine* 328 (1993): 1346–49.

16. K. Johnson, "Ruling by Montana Supreme Court Bolsters Physician-Assisted Suicide," *New York Times,* January 1, 2010, p. A16; *Baxter v. Montana,* No. 2009 MT 449 (Mont. 2009).

17. N. S. Jecker and L. J. Schneiderman, "An Ethical Analysis of the Use of 'Futility' in the 1992 AHA Guidelines for CPR and ECC," *Archives of Internal Medicine* 153 (1993): 2195–98.

18. M. Z. Solomon, L. O'Donnell, and B. Jennings, "Decisions near the End of Life: Professional Views on Life-Sustaining Treatments," *American Journal of Public Health* 83 (1993): 14–23.

19. L. Edelstein, "The Hippocratic Physician," in *Ancient Medicine: Selected Papers of Ludwig Edelstein,* ed. O. Temkin and C. L. Temkin (Baltimore: Johns Hopkins Press, 1967), p. 106.

20. L. J. Schneiderman, *Embracing Our Mortality: Hard Choices in an Age of Medical Miracles* (New York: Oxford University Press, 2008).

21. Yankelovich, *Coming to Public Judgment,* p. 240.

CHAPTER NINE: The Way It Is Now: For Health Professionals

1. F. L. Ferreira, D. P. Bota, A. Bross, C. Mélot, and J. L. Vincent, "Serial Evaluation of the SOFA Score to Predict Outcome in Critically Ill Patients," *JAMA* 286 (2001): 1754–58; J. E. Zimmerman, A. A. Kramer, D. S. McNair, and F. M. Malila, "Acute Physiology and Chronic Health Evaluation (APACHE) IV: Hospital Mortality Assessment for Today's Critically Ill Patient," *Critical Care Medicine* 34 (2006): 1297–1310.

2. R. Macklin, *Enemies of Patients* (New York: Oxford University Press, 1993).

3. Perhaps the most outrageous example of this attitude was the boast of the chief executive of the Ronald Reagan U.C.L.A. Medical Center: "If you come into this hospital, we're not going to let you die." Reported in R. Abelson, "Weighing Medical Costs of End-of-Life Care," *New York Times,* December 23, 2009.

4. J. B. McKinlay, "From Promising Report to Standard Procedure: Seven Stages in the Career of a Medical Innovation," *Milbank Memorial Fund Quarterly / Health and Society* 59 (1981): 383.

5. *Grace Plaza of Great Neck, Inc. v. Elbaum,* 183 A.D. 2d 10, 588 N.Y.S. 2d 853 (1992).

6. D. M. Eddy, "Medicine, Money, and Mathematics," *American College of Surgery Bulletin* 77 (1992): 41, 43.

7. D. A. Grimes, "Technology Follies," *JAMA* 269 (1993): 3030.

8. S. C. Schoenbaum, "Towards Fewer Procedures and Better Outcomes," *JAMA* 269 (1993): 795.

9. S. Miles, "Medical Futility," *Law, Medicine, and Health Care* 20 (1992): 312.

10. L. K. Altman, "Drug Mixture Curbs HIV in Lab, Doctors Report, but Urge Caution," *New York Times*, February 18, 1993, p. Al.

11. K. E. Lasser, P. D. Allen, S. J. Woolhandler, D. U. Himmelstein, S. M. Wolfe, and D. H. Bor, "Timing of New Black Box Warnings and Withdrawals for Prescription Medications," *JAMA* 287 (2002): 2215–20; T. J. Moore, M. R. Cohen, and C. D. Furberg, "Serious Adverse Drug Events Reported to the Food and Drug Administration, 1998–2005," *Archives of Internal Medicine* 167 (2007): 1752–59.

12. T. C. Chalmers, "Ethical Aspects of Clinical Trials," *American Journal of Ophthalmology* 79 (1975): 753–58.

13. Ibid.

14. M. Z. Solomon, L. O'Donnell, B. Jennings, et al., "Decisions near the End of Life: Professional Views of Life-Sustaining Treatments," *American Journal of Public Health* 82 (1993): 14–25.

15. J. M. Wilkinson, "Moral Distress in Nursing Practice: Experience and Effect," *Nursing Forum* 23 (1987–88): 20–21.

16. Chalmers, "Ethical Aspects of Clinical Trials."

17. "University Group Diabetes Program: A Study of the Effects of Hypoglycemic Agents on Vascular Complications in Patients with Adult-Onset Diabetes," *Diabetes* 19, suppl. 2 (1970): 747; P. H. Wang, J. Lau, and T. C. Chalmers, "Meta-Analysis of Effects of Intensive Blood-Glucose Control on Late Complications of Type I Diabetes," *Lancet* 341 (1993): 1306–9; Diabetes Control and Complications Trial Research Group, "The Effect of Intensive Treatment of Diabetes on the Development and Progression of Long-Term Complications in Insulin-Dependent Diabetes Mellitus," *New England Journal of Medicine* 329 (1993): 977–86; P. Reichard, B. Nilsson, and U. Rosenquist, "The Effect of Long-Term Intensified Insulin Treatment on the Development of Microvascular Complications of Diabetes Mellitus," ibid. 329 (1993): 304–9; H. C. Gerstein, M. E. Miller, R. P. Byington, et al. (Action to Control Cardiovascular Risk in Diabetes Study Group), "Effects of Intensive Glucose Lowering in Type 2 Diabetes," ibid. 358 (2008): 2545–59; W. Duckworth, C. Abraira, T. Moritz, et al. (VADT Investigators), "Glucose Control and Vascular Complications in Veterans with Type 2 Diabetes," ibid. 360 (2009): 129–39; A. Patel, S. MacMahon, J. Chalmers, et al. (ADVANCE Collaborative Group), "Intensive Blood Glucose Control and Vascular Outcomes in Patients with Type 2 Diabetes," ibid. 358 (2008): 2560–72; T. N. Kelly, L. A. Bazzano, V. A. Fonseca, T. K. Theti, K. Reynolds, and J. He, "Systematic Review: Glucose Control and Cardiovascular Disease in Type 2 Diabetes," *Annals of Internal Medicine* 151 (2009): 394–403; R. S. Wiener, D. C. Wiener, and R. J. Larson, "Benefits and Risks of Tight Glucose Control in Critically Ill Adults: A Meta-Analysis," *JAMA* 300 (2008): 933–44.

18. E. F. Unger, A. M. Thompson, M. J. K. Blank, and R. Temple, "Erythropoiesis-Stimulating Agents: Time for a Reevaluation," *New England Journal of Medicine* 362 (2010): 189–92.

19. Schoenbaum, "Towards Fewer Procedures and Better Outcomes."

20. Ibid.

21. G. Kolata, "Mammogram Debate Took Group Off Guard," *New York Times*, November 20, 2009, p. A22; R. Aronowitz, "Addicted to Mammograms," *New York Times*, November 20, 2009, p. A31.

22. G. A. Diamond and T. A. Denton, "Alternative Perspectives on the Biased Foundations of Medical Technology Assessment," *Annals of Internal Medicine* 118 (1993): 455–64.

23. D. Gesensway, "Building a Better Clinical Practice Guideline: Conquering Bias Remains a Key Challenge," *ACP Observer* 13, no. 6 (1993): 1.

24. B. G. Charlton, "Public Health Medicine: A Different Kind of Ethics?" *Journal of the Royal Society of Medicine* 86 (1993): 194.

25. Kolata, "Mammogram Debate Took Group Off Guard"; Aronowitz, "Addicted to Mammograms."

26. L. J. Schneiderman, R. M. Kaplan, R. A. Pearlman, and H. Teetzel, "Do Physicians' Own Preferences for Life-Sustaining Treatment Influence Their Perceptions of Patients' Preferences?" *Journal of Clinical Ethics* 4 (1993): 28–33.

27. R. F. Uhlmann, R. A. Pearlman, and K. C. Cain, "Physicians' and Spouses' Predictions of Elderly Patients' Resuscitation Preferences," *Journal of Gerontology* 43, no. 5 (1988): 115–21.

28. Schneiderman et al., "Do Physicians' Own Preferences for Life-Sustaining Treatment Influence Their Perceptions of Patients' Preferences?"

29. M. J. Barry, quoted in J. F. Kasper, A. G. Mulley, and J. E. Wennberg, "Developing Shared Decision-Making Programs to Improve the Quality of Health Care," *Quality Review Bulletin* 18 (1992): 183–90.

30. G. Kolata, "Though Results are Unproved, Robotic Surgery Wins Converts," *New York Times*, February 14, 2010, pp. 1, 19.

31. D. Leonhardt, "Finding the Nerve to Cut Costs," *New York Times*, December 9, 2009, p. B1.

32. D. Leonhardt, "Where Cuts Haven't Hurt Patients," *New York Times*, December 30, 2009, p. B1.

33. A. Langer, quoted in G. Kolata, "Mammogram Debate Moving from Test's Merits to Its Cost," *New York Times*, December 27, 1993, p. A1.

34. D. Grady, "Study Questions Safety of Mammograms for Young Women at High Risk of Cancer," *New York Times*, December 1, 2009.

35. A. Meisel, "Legal Consensus about Forgoing Life-Sustaining Treatment: Its Status and Its Prospects," *Kennedy Institute of Ethics Journal 2* (1992): 333.

36. E. Eckholm, "Those Who Pay Health Costs Think about Drawing Lines," *New York Times*, March 28, 1993, sec. 4, p. 1.

37. Ibid.

38. J. E. Brody, "Personal Health: The Rights of a Dying Patient Are Often Misunderstood, Even by Medical Professionals," *New York Times*, January 27, 1993, p. B7.

39. D. M. Mirvis, "Physicians' Autonomy: The Relation between Public and Professional Expectations," *New England Journal of Medicine* 328 (1993): 1347.

40. J. D. Lantos, P. A. Singer, R. M. Walker, et al., "The Illusion of Futility in Clinical Practice," *American Journal of Medicine* 87 (1989): 81–84; T. Brennan, "Right-to-Die Dilemma: Are Ethics Committees Equipped to Fill Their Roles?" *American Medical News*, November 11 (1991): 28; A. M. Capron, "In re Helga Wanglie," *Hastings Center Report* 21,

no. 5 (1991): 26–28; D. Callahan, "Medical Futility, Medical Necessity: The Problem-without-a-Name," *Hastings Center Report* 21, no. 4 (1991): 30–35, respectively.

41. President's Commission for the Study of Ethical Problems in Medicine and Bio-medical and Behavioral Research, *Deciding to Forgo Life-Sustaining Treatment: Ethical, Medical, and Legal Issues in Treatment Decisions* (Washington, DC: Government Printing Office, 1983); *Guidelines on the Termination of Life-Sustaining Treatment and the Care of the Dying* (Briarcliff Manor, NY: Hastings Center, 1987); Council on Ethical and Judicial Affairs, *Current Opinions* (Chicago: Council on Ethical and Judicial Affairs of the American Medical Association, 1989); Task Force on Ethics of the Society of Critical Care Medicine, "Consensus Report on the Ethics of Forgoing Life-Sustaining Treatments in the Critically Ill," *Critical Care Medicine* 18 (1990): 1435–39; American Thoracic Society, "Withholding and Withdrawing Life-Sustaining Therapy," *Annals of Internal Medicine* 115 (1991): 478–85; AMA-YPS Handbook Review: HOD Reference Committee on Amendments to Constitution and Bylaws, www.amaassn.org/ama1/pub/upload/mm/17/gridcandb.pdf.

42. N. S. Jecker and L. J. Schneiderman, "Futility and Rationing," *American Journal of Medicine* 92 (1992): 189–96.

43. President's Commission for the Study of Ethical Problems in Medicine and Bio-medical and Behavioral Research, *Defining Death* (Washington, DC: Government Printing Office, 1981); "Guidelines for the Determination of Death," *JAMA* 246 (1981): 2184–86.

44. D. Rennie and A. Flanagin, "Publication Bias: The Triumph of Hope over Experience," *JAMA* 267 (1992): 411–12.

45. F. L. Ferreira, et al., "Serial Evaluation of the SOFA Score to Predict Outcome in Critically Ill Patients," *JAMA* 286 (2001): 1754–58; Zimmerman et al. "Acute Physiology and Chronic Health Evaluation (APACHE) IV"; M. M. Pollack, U. E. Ruttimann, and P. R. Getson, "The Pediatric Risk of Mortality (PRISM) Score," *Critical Care Medicine* 16 (1988): 1110–16; R. W. S. Chang, "Individual Outcome Prediction Models for Intensive Care Units," *Lancet* 2, no. 8655 (1989): 143–46; U. E. Ruttimann and M. M. Pollack, "Objective Assessment of Changing Mortality Risks in Pediatric Intensive Care Unit Patients," *Critical Care Medicine* 19 (1991): 474–83; U. E. Ruttimann and M. M. Pollack, "A Time-Series Approach to Outcome Prediction," *Computers and Biomedical Research* 26 (1993): 353–72; Task Force of the American College of Critical Care Medicine, "Guidelines for Intensive Care Unit Admission, Discharge, and Triage," *Critical Care Medicine* 27 (1999): 633–38.

46. C. Sasson, A. L. Kellermann, and B. F. McNally, "Prehospital Termination of Resuscitation in Cases of Refractory Out-of-Hospital Cardiac Arrest," *JAMA* 300 (2008): 1432–38.

47. L. J. Schneiderman, N. S. Jecker, and A. R. Jonsen, "Medical Futility: Its Meaning and Ethical Implications," *Annals of Internal Medicine* 112 (1990): 949–54.

48. Emergency Cardiac Care Committee and Subcommittees, American Heart Association, "Guidelines for Cardiopulmonary Resuscitation and Emergency Cardiac Care, VII: Ethical Considerations in Resuscitation," *JAMA* 268 (1992): 2282–88; N. S. Jecker and L. J. Schneiderman, "Ceasing Futile Resuscitation in the Field: Ethical Considerations," *Archives of Internal Medicine* 152 (1992): 2392–97; N. S. Jecker and L. J. Schneiderman, "An Ethical Analysis of the Use of 'Futility' in the 1992 American Heart Association Guidelines for Cardiopulmonary Resuscitation and Emergency Cardiac Care," *Archives of Internal Medicine* 153 (1993): 2195–98; K. M. McIntyre, "Loosening Criteria

for Withholding Prehospital Cardiopulmonary Resuscitation," *Archives of Internal Medicine* 153 (1993): 2189–92.

49. Emergency Cardiac Care Committee and Subcommittees, "Guidelines for Cardiopulmonary Resuscitation."

50. Sasson, Kellermann, and McNally, "Prehospital Termination of Resuscitation."

51. J. H. King, The *Law of Medical Malpractice in a Nutshell* (St. Paul: West Publishing, 1977), pp. 42–49; J. H. King, "In Search of a Standard of Care for the Medical Profession: The 'Accepted Practice' Formula," *Vanderbilt Law Review* 28 (1975): 1213–76.

52. M. B. Kapp, " 'Cookbook' Medicine: A Legal Perspective," *Archives of Internal Medicine* 150 (1990): 496–500.

53. L. K. Stell, "Stopping Treatment on Grounds of Futility: A Role for Institutional Policy," *St. Louis University Public Law Review* 11 (1992): 481–97.

54. Schneiderman, Jecker, and Jonsen, "Medical Futility."

55. A. L. Kellermann D. R. Staves, and B. B. Hackman, "In-Hospital Resuscitation Following Unsuccessful Prehospital Advanced Cardiac Life Support: 'Heroic Efforts' or an Exercise in Futility?" *Annals of Emergency Medicine* 17 (1988): 589–94; J. D. Lantos, S. H. Miles, M. D. Silverstein, and C. B. Stocking, "Survival after Cardiopulmonary Resuscitation in Babies of Very Low Birthweight: Is CPR Futile?" *New England Journal of Medicine* 318 (1988): 91–95; G. E. Taffet, T. A. Teasdale, and R. J. Luchi, "In-Hospital Cardiopulmonary Resuscitation," *JAMA* 260 (1988): 2069–72; D. J. Murphy, A. M. Murray, B. E. Robinson, and E. W. Campion, "Outcomes of Cardiopulmonary Resuscitation in the Elderly," *Annals of Internal Medicine* 111 (1989): 199–205; M. J. Bonnin and R. A. Swor, "Outcomes in Unsuccessful Field Resuscitation Attempts," *Annals of Emergency Medicine* 18 (1989): 507–12; K. Faber-Langendoen, "Resuscitation of Patients with Metastatic Cancer: Is Transient Benefit Still Futile?" *Archives of Internal Medicine* 151 (1991): 235–39; W. A. Gray, R. J. Capone, and A. S. Most, "Unsuccessful Emergency Medical Resuscitation: Are Continued Efforts in the Emergency Department Justified?" *New England Journal of Medicine* 329 (1991): 1393–98.

56. M. Rosenberg, C. Wang, S. Hoffman-Wilde, and D. Hickham, "Results of Cardiopulmonary Resuscitation: Failure to Predict Survival in Two Community Hospitals," *Archives of Internal Medicine* 153 (1993): 1370–75.

57. AMA-YPS Handbook Review: HOD Reference Committee on Amendments to Constitution and Bylaws.

58. "Uniform Health-Care Decisions Act," Drafted by the National Conference of Commissioners on Uniform State Laws, Approved and Recommended for Enactment in All the States, Charleston, SC, July 30–August 6, 1993, Prefatory Note 5. Available from National Conference of Commissioners on Uniform State Laws, 676 North St. Clair Street, Suite 1700, Chicago, IL 60611.

59. Ibid., section 7: Obligations of Health-Care Provider, subsection f.

60. L. J. Schneiderman and N. S. Jecker, "Futility in Practice," *Archives of Internal Medicine* 153 (1993): 437–41.

61. "At Odds with Family, Hospital Seeks to End Life," *Chicago Tribune,* January 10, 1991; "Atlanta Court Bars Efforts to End Life Support for Stricken Girl, 13," *New York Times,* October 18, 1991; D. Gianelli, "Hospital Seeks to Override Family's Objections, Stop Respirator," *American Medical News,* Jan. 28, 1992, sec. 2; L. Belkin, "As Family Protests, Hospital Seeks an End to Woman's Life Support," *New York Times,* January 10, 1991, p. A1.

62. *In the Matter of Baby "K,"* 16 F.3d F. Supp. 590 (E.D. Va. 1993); WL 38674 (4th Cir. 1994).

63. L. J. Schneiderman and A. M. Capron, "How Can Hospital Futility Policies Contribute to Establishing Standards of Practice?" *Cambridge Quarterly of Healthcare Ethics* 9 (2000): 524–31.

CHAPTER TEN: The High Points

1. *In the Matter of Baby "K"* (The Baby K Case), 832 F. Supp. 1022 (E.D. Va. 1993): WL 343557.

2. *In the Matter of Baby "K,"* 16 F.3d F. Supp. 590 (E.D. VA 1993). WL 38674 (4th Cir. 1994).

3. Emergency Medical Treatment and Active Labor Act (EMTALA), 42 U.S.C.A. #139dd (West 1992).

4. Americans with Disabilities Act, Public Law No. 101–336 (July 26, 1990).

5. L. J. Schneiderman and S. Manning, "The Baby K Case: A Search for the Elusive Standard of Medical Care," *Cambridge Quarterly of Healthcare Ethics* 6 (1997): 9–18.

6. *Bryan v. Rectors and Visitors of the University of Virginia*, 95 F.3d 349 (4th Cir. 1996).

7. L. J. Schneiderman, N. S. Jecker, and A. R. Jonsen, "Medical Futility: Its Meaning and Ethical Implications," *Annals of Internal Medicine* 112 (1990): 949–54.

8. J. D. Lantos, P. A. Singer, R. M. Walter, et al., "The Illusion of Futility in Clinical Practice," *American Journal of Medicine* 87 (1989): 81–84; S. J. Youngner, "Who Defines Futility?" *JAMA* 260 (1988): 2094–95.

9. J. J. Paris, M. D. Schreiber, M. Statter, R. Arensman, and M. Siegler, "Beyond Autonomy: Physicians' Refusal to Use Life-Prolonging Extracorporeal Membrane Oxygenation," *New England Journal of Medicine* 329 (1993): 356.

10. D. W. Amundsen, "The Physician's Obligation to Prolong Life: A Medical Duty without Classical Roots," *Hastings Center Report* 8, no. 4 (1978): 23–30.

11. B. Jennett and F. Plum, "Persistent Vegetative State after Brain Damage: A Syndrome in Search of a Name," *Lancet* 1 (1972): 734–37.

12. R. D. Truog, A. S. Brett, and J. Frader, "The Problem with Futility," *New England Journal of Medicine* 326 (1992): 1560–64.

13. President's Commission for the Study for Ethical Problems in Medicine and Biomedical and Behavioral Research, *Deciding to Forgo Life-Sustaining Treatment: Ethical, Medical, and Legal Issues in Treatment Decisions* (Washington, DC: Government Printing Office, 1983); *Guidelines on the Termination of Life-Sustaining Treatment and the Care of the Dying* (Briarcliff Manor, NY: Hastings Center, 1987); Council on Ethical and Judicial Affairs, *Current Opinions* (Chicago: Council on Ethical and Judicial Affairs, American Medical Association, 1989); Task Force on Ethics of the Society of Critical Care Medicine, "Consensus Report on the Ethics of Forgoing Life-Sustaining Treatments in the Critically Ill," *Critical Care Medicine* 18 (1990): 1435–39; American Thoracic Society, "Withholding and Withdrawing Life-Sustaining Therapy," *Annals of Internal Medicine* 115 (1991): 478–85.

14. Truog, Brett, and Frader, "The Problem with Futility."

15. D. Postema, personal communication.

16. Hippocratic Corpus, "The Art," in *Ethics in Medicine: Historical Perspectives and*

Contemporary Concerns, ed. S. J. Reiser, A. J. Dyck, and W. J. Curran (Cambridge: MIT Press, 1977), pp. 6–7.

17. Plato, *Republic,* trans. G. M. A. Grube (Indianapolis: Hackett Publishing, 1981), pp. 76–77.

18. Schneiderman, Jecker, and Jonsen, "Medical Futility: Its Meaning."

19. A. L. Kellermann, D. R. Staves, and B. B. Hackman, "In-Hospital Resuscitation Following Unsuccessful Prehospital Advanced Cardiac Life-Support: 'Heroic Efforts' or an Exercise in Futility?" *Annals of Emergency Medicine* 17 (1988): 589–94; J. D. Lantos, S. H. Miles, M. D. Silverstein, and C. B. Stocking, "Survival after Cardiopulmonary Resuscitation in Babies of Very Low Birth Weight: Is CPR Futile?" *New England Journal of Medicine* 318 (1988): 91–95; G. E. Taffet, T. A. Teasdale, and R. J. Luchi, "In-Hospital Cardiopulmonary Resuscitation," *JAMA* 260 (1988): 2069–72; D. J. Murphy, A. M. Murray, B. E. Robinson, et al., "Outcomes of Cardiopulmonary Resuscitation in the Elderly," *Annals of Internal Medicine* (1989): 199–205; M. J. Bonnin and R. A. Swor, "Outcomes in Unsuccessful Field Resuscitation Attempts," *Annals of Emergency Medicine* 18 (1989): 507–12; K. Faber-Langendoen, "Resuscitation of Patients with Metastatic Cancer: Is Transient Benefit Still Futile?" *Archives of Internal Medicine* 151 (1991): 235–39; W. A. Gray, R. J. Capone, and A. S. Most, "Unsuccessful Emergency Medical Resuscitation: Are Continued Efforts in the Emergency Department Justified?" *New England Journal of Medicine* 329 (1991): 1393–98.

20. N. S. Jecker and L. J. Schneiderman, "Medical Futility: The Duty Not to Treat," *Cambridge Quarterly of Healthcare Ethics 2* (1993): 151–57.

21. L. J. Schneiderman and A. M. Capron, "How Can Hospital Futility Policies Contribute to Establishing Standards of Practice?" *Cambridge Quarterly of Healthcare Ethics* 9 (2000): 524–31.

22. Ibid.

23. T. Tomlinson and H. Brody, "Futility and the Ethics of Resuscitation," *JAMA* 264 (1990): 1276–80.

24. Truog, Brett, and Frader, "The Problem with Futility."

25. L. J. Schneiderman and N. S. Jecker, "Futility in Practice," *Archives of Internal Medicine* 153 (1993): 437–41.

26. N. S. Jecker and L. J. Schneiderman, "Futility and Rationing," *American Journal of Medicine* 92 (1992): 189–96.

27. L. J. Schneiderman, K. Faber-Langendoen, and N. S. Jecker, "Beyond Futility to an Ethic of Care," *American Journal of Medicine* 96 (1994): 110–14.

28. H. Brody, M. L. Campbell, K. Faber-Langendoen, and K.S. Ogle, "Withdrawing Intensive Life-Sustaining Treatment: Recommendations for Compassionate Clinical Management," *New England Journal of Medicine* 336 (1997): 652–57; D. E. Weissman, "Decision Making at a Time of Crisis near the End of Life," *JAMA* 292 (2004): 1738–43; R. A. Mularski, J. R. Curtis, J. A. Billings, et al., "Proposed Quality Measures for Palliative Care in the Critically Ill: A Consensus from the Robert Wood Johnson Foundation Critical Care Workgroup," *Critical Care Medicine* 34, no. 11, Suppl. (2006): S404–11.

29. M. K. Tamura, K. E. Covinsky, G. M. Chertow, K. Yaffe, S. Landefeld, and C. E. McCulloch, "Functional Status of Elderly Adults before and after Initiation of Dialysis," *New England Journal of Medicine* 361 (2009): 1539–47.

30. S. L. Mitchell, J. M. Teno, D. K. Kiely, et al., "The Clinical Course of Advanced Dementia," *New England Journal of Medicine* 361 (2009): 1529–38.

CHAPTER ELEVEN: Medical Futility

1. L. J. Schneiderman, N. S. Jecker, and A. R. Jonsen, "Medical Futility: Its Meaning and Ethical Implications," *Annals of Internal Medicine* 112 (1990): 949–54.

2. L. J. Schneiderman, N. S. Jecker, and A. R. Jonsen, "Medical Futility: Response to Critiques," *Annals of Internal Medicine* 125 (1996): 669–774.

3. S. M. Wolf, "Conflict between Doctor and Patient," *Law, Medicine and Health Care* 16 (1988): 197–203.

4. G. R. Scofield, "Medical Futility: Can We Talk?" *Generations* 18, no. 4 (1994): 66–70; R. M. Veatch and C. M. Spicer, "Medically Futile Care: The Role of the Physician in Setting Limits," *American Journal of Law and Medicine* 18 (1992): 15–36; T. A. Brennan, "Silent Decisions: Limits of Consent and the Terminally Ill Patient," *Law Medicine and Health Care* 16 (1988): 204–9; G. R. Scofield, "Is Consent Useful When Resuscitation Isn't?" *Hastings Center Report* 21, no. 6 (1991): 28–36.

5. T. J. Prendergast, "Futility and the Common Cold: How Requests for Antibiotics Can Illuminate Care at the End of Life," *Chest* 107 (1995): 836–44; Scofield, "Medical Futility."

6. D. J. Murphy, "Do-Not-Resuscitate Orders: Time for Reappraisal in Long-Term-Care Institutions," *JAMA* 260 (1988): 2098–2101; H. Brody, "Medical Futility: A Useful Concept?" in *Medical Futility*, ed. M. Zucker and H. Zucker (New York: Cambridge University Press, 1996); J. J. Paris, R. K. Crone, and F. Reardon, "Physician's Refusal of Requested Treatment: The Case of Baby L," *New England Journal of Medicine* 322 (1990): 1012–15; H. Brody, "The Power to Determine Futility," chap. 11 in *The Healer's Power* (New Haven, CT: Yale University Press, 1992).

7. Brody, "The Power to Determine Futility"; N. S. Jecker, "Medical Futility and Care of the Dying Patient," *Western Journal of Medicine* 163 (1995): 287–91; N. S. Jecker and R. A. Pearlman, "Medical Futility: Who Decides?" *Archives of Internal Medicine* 152 (1992): 1140–44; N. S. Jecker, "Is Refusal of Futile Treatment Unjustified Paternalism?" *Journal of Clinical Ethics* 6 (1995): 130–44.

8. Veatch and Spicer, "Medically Futile Care."

9. N. S. Jecker and L. J. Schneiderman, "When Families Request That Everything Possible Be Done," *Journal of Medicine and Philosophy* 20 (1995): 145–63; L. J. Schneiderman, K. Faber-Langendoen, and N. S. Jecker, "Beyond Futility to an Ethic of Care," *American Journal of Medicine* 96 (1994): 110–14.

10. R. D. Truog, A. S. Brett, and J. Frader, "The Problem with Futility," *New England Journal of Medicine* 326 (1992): 1560–64; E. H. Morreim, "Profoundly Diminished Life: The Casualties of Coercion," *Hastings Center Report* 24, no. 1 (1994): 33–42; S. J. Youngner, "Medical Futility and the social contract (Who Are the Real Doctors on Howard Brody's Island?)," *Seton Hall Law Review* 25 (1995): 1015–26; R. A. Gatter and J. C. Moskop, "From Futility to Triage," *Journal of Medicine and Philosophy* 20 (1995): 191–205.

11. J. R. Curtis, D. R. Park, M. R. Krone, and R. A. Pearlman, "The Use of the Medical Futility Rationale in Do Not Attempt Resuscitation Orders," *JAMA* 273 (1995): 124–28; S. V. Van McCrary, J. W. Swanson, S. J. Youngner, H. S. Perkins, and W. J. Winslade, "Physicians' Quantitative Assessments of Medical Futility," *Journal of Clinical Ethics* 5 (1994): 100–105.

12. D. Yankelovich, *Coming to Public Judgment: Making Democracy Work in a Complex World* (Syracuse, NY: Syracuse University Press, 1991).

13. Wolf, "Conflict between Doctor and Patient"; Brennan, "Silent Decisions"; Truog, Brett, and Frader, "The Problem with Futility"; F. Ackerman, "The Significance of a Wish," *Hastings Center Report* 21, no. 4 (1991): 27–29; A. M. Capron, "In re Helga Wanglie," ibid. 21, no. 5 (1991): 26–28.

14. G. Kolata, "Court Ruling Limits Rights of Patients: Care Deemed Futile May Be Withheld," *New York Times*, April 22, 1995, p. 6; N. S. Jecker, "Calling It Quits: Stopping Futile Treatment and Caring for Patients," *Journal of Clinical Ethics* 5 (1994): 138–42; L. J. Schneiderman and N. S. Jecker, "Futility in Practice," *Archives of Internal Medicine* 153 (1993): 437–41.

15. *Texas Health and Safety Code, Annotated*, sec. 166.046.

16. "Uniform Health-Care Decisions Act," Drafted by the National Conference of Commissioners on Uniform State Laws, Approved and Recommended for Enactment in All the States, Charleston, SC, July 30–August 6, 1993, Prefatory Note 5. Available from National Conference of Commissioners on Uniform State Laws, 676 North St. Clair Street, Suite 1700, Chicago, IL 60611.

17. Ibid., section 7: Obligations of Health-Care Provider, subsection f.

18. Truog, Brett, and Frader, "The Problem with Futility."

19. Emergency Cardiac Care Committee and Subcommittees, American Heart Association, "Guidelines for Cardiopulmonary Resuscitation and Emergency Cardiac Care, VII: Ethical Consideration in Resuscitation," *JAMA* 268 (1992): 2283; N. S. Jecker and L. J. Schneiderman, "An Ethical Analysis of the Use of Futility in the 1992 American Heart Association Guidelines for CPR and EC," *Archives of Internal Medicine* 153 (1993): 2195–98; N. S. Jecker and L. J. Schneiderman, "Ceasing Futile Resuscitation in the Field: Ethical Considerations," *Archives of Internal Medicine* 152 (1992): 2392–97.

20. L. J. Schneiderman, "The Futility Debate: Effective versus Beneficial Intervention," *Journal of the American Geriatric Society* 42 (1994): 883–86.

21. Scofield, "Is Consent Useful When Resuscitation Isn't?"

22. K. R. Popper, *The Logic of Scientific Discovery* (New York: Basic Books, 1961), p. 280.

23. T. Tomlinson and D. Czlonka, "Futility and Hospital Policy," *Hastings Center Report* 25, no. 3 (1995): 28–35.

24. Schneiderman, Jecker, and Jonsen, "Medical Futility."

25. L. J. Schneiderman and N. S. Jecker, "Is the Treatment Beneficial, Experimental or Futile?" *Cambridge Quarterly of Healthcare Ethics* 5 (1996): 248–56.

26. Prendergast, "Futility and the Common Cold."

27. Schneiderman, Jecker, and Jonsen, "Medical Futility."

28. Prendergast, "Futility and the Common Cold."

29. Emergency Cardiac Care Committee and Subcommittees, American Heart Association, "Guidelines for Cardiopulmonary Resuscitation and Emergency Cardiac Care."

30. Jecker and Schneiderman, "The Use of Futility in the 1992 American Heart Association Guidelines for CPR and EC."

31. Prendergast, "Futility and the Common Cold."

32. J. D. Lantos, S. H. Miles, M. D. Silverstein, and C. B. Stocking, "Survival after Cardiopulmonary Resuscitation in Babies of Very Low Birth Weight: Is CPR Futile?" *New England Journal of Medicine* 318 (1988): 91–95; A. L. Kellermann, D. R. Staves, and B. B. Hackman, "In-Hospital Resuscitation Following Unsuccessful Prehospital Advanced Cardiac Life Support: 'Heroic Efforts' or an Exercise in Futility?" *Annals of Emergency Medicine* 17 (1988): 589–94; M. J. Bonnin and R. A. Swor, "Outcomes in Unsuccessful Field Resuscitation

Attempts," *Annals of Emergency Medicine* 18 (1989): 507–12; D. J. Murphy, A. M. Murray, B. E. Robinson, and E. W. Campion, "Outcomes of Cardiopulmonary Resuscitation in the Elderly," *Annals of Internal Medicine* 111 (1989): 199–105; K. Faber-Langendoen, "Resuscitation of Patients with Metastatic Cancer: Is Transient Benefit Still Futile?" *Archives of Internal Medicine* 151 (1991): 235–39; W. A. Gray, R. J. Capone, and A. S. Most, "Unsuccessful Emergency Medical Resuscitation: Are Continued Efforts in the Emergency Department Justified?" *New England Journal of Medicine* 325 (1991): 1393–98.

33. C. Sasson, A. L. Kellermann, and B. F. McNally, "Prehospital Termination of Resuscitation in Cases of Refractory Out-of-Hospital Cardiac Arrest," *JAMA* 300 (2008): 1432–38.

34. D. A. Grimes, "Technology Follies," *JAMA* 269 (1993): 3030–32.

35. For example, F. L. Ferreira, D. P. Bota, A. Bross, C. Mélot, and J. L. Vincent, "Serial Evaluation of the SOFA Score to Predict Outcome in Critically Ill Patients," *JAMA* 286 (2001): 1754–58; J. E. Zimmerman, A. A. Kramer, D. S. McNair, and F. M. Malila, "Acute Physiology and Chronic Health Evaluation (APACHE) IV: Hospital Mortality Assessment for Today's Critically Ill Patient," *Critical Care Medicine* 34 (2006): 1297–1310.

36. B. A. Brody and A. Halevy, "Is Futility a Futile Concept?" *Journal of Medicine and Philosophy* 20 (1995): 123–44.

37. S. G. Post, "Baby K: Medical Futility and the Free Exercise of Religion," *Journal of Law, Medicine, and Ethics* 23 (1995): 20–26.

38. N. S. Jecker, J. A. Carrese, and R. A. Pearlman, "Caring for Patients in Cross-Cultural Settings," *Hastings Center Report* 25, no. 1 (1995): 6–14.

39. E. H. Morreim, *Balancing Act: The New Medical Ethics of Medicine's New Economics* (Boston: Kulwer Academic Publishers, 1991).

40. N. S. Jecker and L. J. Schneiderman, "Futility and Rationing," *American Journal of Medicine* 92 (1992): 189–96; L. J. Schneiderman and N. S. Jecker, "Should a Criminal Receive a Heart Transplant? Medical Justice vs. Societal Justice," *Theoretical Medicine,* June 1995.

41. H. Brody, "The Physician's Role in Determining Futility," *Journal of the American Geriatrics Society* 42 (1994): 875–78.

42. Truog, Brett, and Frader, "The Problem with Futility."

43. Hippocratic Corpus, "The Art," in *Ethics in Medicine: Historical Perspectives and Contemporary Concerns,* ed. S. J. Reiser, A. J. Dyck, and W. J. Curran (Cambridge: MIT Press, 1977), p. 6.

44. N. S. Jecker, "Knowing When to Stop: The Limits of Medicine," *Hastings Center Report* May-June (1991): 5–8.

45. Schneiderman, Jecker, and Jonsen, "Medical Futility."

46. *Texas Health and Safety Code, Annotated,* sec. 166.046. This statute provides specific guidelines for resolving disputes around decisions to forgo futile treatments. It requires the involvement of all interested parties, from the patient's perspective as well as that of expert medical specialists and the ethics committee. Hence, reasons for forgoing life-prolonging treatment are critically evaluated.

47. L. J. Schneiderman, *Embracing Our Mortality: Hard Choices in an Age of Medical Miracles* (New York: Oxford University Press, 2008).

Index

abortion, 6–7, 12, 13, 54, 108, 112, 176; and Catholic hospitals, 126, 191; and public opinion, 137; and respect for life, 134, 135
advance directive, 97, 99, 100–101
age, x, 47–48, 55, 80–81, 85. *See also* child; elderly people
AIDS, 35, 45, 149. *See also* human immunodeficiency virus (HIV) infection
Alicia M. (case study), 24–25, 27, 28
Alzheimer's disease, 35, 182
American Academy of Neurology, 40
American Academy of Pediatrics, 168
American College of Obstetricians and Gynecologists, 92
American College of Physicians, 154
American Heart Association (AHA), 40, 138, 154, 161, 188
American Medical Association, xi, 40, 138, 164, 185–86; Code of Medical Ethics, 164; Council on Ethical and Judicial Affairs, 117
American Nurses' Association, 40
Americans with Disabilities Act (ADA), 165, 168, 206n38
American Thoracic Society, 40, 138
anencephaly, 41, 84, 105, 141, 163, 165, 167–69, 206n38
Annas, George, 3
APACHE (Acute Physiology, Age, Chronic Health Evaluation), 159
Aristotle, 33
athletes, 10–11, 16, 170

Baby K, 41, 84, 105, 167–69, 206n38
Bacon, Francis, 7
Barber v. Los Angeles County Superior Court, 40, 98
Basic Life Support Rule (BLS), 17, 189

Bauby, Jean-Dominique, 120
benefit, 10, 38, 39; and burdens, 97–98, 110; and effects, 152, 168; and harm, 10, 157; and risks, 158; small, 139
bioethics, 3, 45, 154–55
biological existence, 14, 19, 95, 111, 122, 161. *See also* body; physiology
biomedical ethical organizations, 116–17
body, 11, 13, 16, 19, 146, 164; effects on, 152, 154, 171; and person, 9. *See also* biological existence; life; physiology
bone marrow transplantation, 51, 74, 75, 76, 94
Boxley, Mrs. (case study), 37–39, 40, 47–48, 52, 53, 55
brain, 1–2, 3, 58, 59, 62, 63; and criteria for death, 8, 14, 85–86, 128, 159, 185; hemorrhage of, 174; irreversible damage to, 117; and Linares, 89–90; patient's knowledge about, 101; recovery of, 4. *See also* anencephaly; unconsciousness, permanent; vegetative state, permanent
Bryan v. Rectors and Visitors of the University of Virginia, 216n6
Bush, George H. W., 54
Bush, Jeb, 62

California Appellate Court, 40
California Medical Association, 164
California Supreme Court, x, 102
Camus, Albert, 21
cancer, 45, 52, 92, 152, 182; breast, 94, 156–57; and CPR, 50; and renal dialysis, 79
cardiopulmonary resuscitation (CPR), xi, 21, 106, 178; and Baby K, 167; benefit vs. harm from, 112–13; effectiveness of, 52; empirical data on, 174; as extraordinary vs. ordinary,

cardiopulmonary resuscitation (CPR) *(cont.)*
97; likelihood of success of, 16–17, 163; and
metastatic cancer, 107–8, 109, 182; patient's
knowledge about, 101; on patients unlikely
to survive, 49–50; standards for attempting,
161–62; withholding of, 79–80, 82, 187–88
care: and emotional connections, 68–69; ethic
of, 68–72, 73, 87, 180–81; medically beneficial, 16; misguided understanding of, 21; as
never futile, x, 8, 19; palliative, 69, 72, 99,
132; provision of, 114; right to basic, 45; and
treatment, x; and women, 69. *See also* comfort care
Cather, Willa, 29, 55–56
Catholic Church, 6–7, 99, 123, 134
Catholic hospitals, 191
Catholicism, 97, 124, 125, 126. *See also* Christianity
cesarean delivery, 92, 93
child: death of, 24–25, 28–29, 31, 32–34; grati-
tude for life of, 33; pain of losing, 64; severely
disabled, 54. *See also* age
Christianity, 6, 99, 122–23, 134. *See also*
Catholicism; religion
Clinton, Bill, ix
comfort care, 20, 68, 70, 87, 114, 145, 181; and
Alicia M., 24; as appropriate, 185; and Boxley,
38; defined, 18–19; duty to provide, 71; inter-
ference with, 31; for patient vs. family, 28; in
terminal stages, 21; total context for, 72. *See
also* care
common sense, 9, 19, 41, 106, 116, 118, 162,
174
communication, 31, 32, 70–71, 100
community, 39, 54, 119, 155
compassion, 21, 31, 32, 38, 157, 158, 178
conflict-of-interest, 46, 60, 93
Congress, 45, 46, 48, 79, 186; Office of Technology Assessment, 147. *See also* legislation
cost, 76, 83, 142; and beneficial treatment, 140;
and benefits vs. burdens criterion, 97; of care
six months before death, 80; of care taken
from others, 128; of comfort and palliative
care, 180; containment of, 87, 127–28, 159,
191; and defensive medicine, 92; of drugs,
50; and economic limitations, 142; and
elderly people, 80, 81; factors contributing

to, 44–48; and finite resources, 116; and need
for care standards, 169; and permanent vegetative state, 47; for renal dialysis, 48–49; rising, 77; of technology, 45, 78, 156; and treatment variations, 148
Council of the American Recovery and Reinvestment Act (ARRA), 45–46
courts, 22, 42, 55, 101–3, 141; and Baby K, 168;
and Cruzan, 2; and fraudulent treatments,
92–93; guidelines for, 166; idiosyncratic decisions of, 165; and Linares, 90, 147; and Schiavo, 63; termination of life support as requiring, 99–100; and Wanglie case, 59, 60. *See
also* lawsuit; litigation
Cruzan, Joe, 2
Cruzan, Nancy, 7, 42, 54, 57, 170; appreciation
of treatment by, 17; and body vs. person, 9;
dignity and respect for, 12–13; and distortion
of medical goals, 22; and effects vs. benefits,
12; permanent unconsciousness of, 1–3
Cruzan family, 5, 41, 54, 101, 102
Cruzan v. Director, Missouri Department of Health,
2, 39, 96, 97, 99, 104

Daniels, Norman, 63, 64
Daubert v. Merrell Dow, 93
death, 19, 80, 106; acceptance of, 22, 25–26,
87, 129, 185; age at, 32–33, 34; blame for, 26;
and brain function, 8, 14, 85–86, 128, 159,
185; of child, 31, 32–34; communication
about, 52; definition of, 159, 185; denial of,
64, 70–71; as evil, 26, 32, 128–29; as exceed-
ing medical powers, 9; and experimental
treatments, 149; with family and friends,
70, 72; and family loss, 65; fear of, 128, 129;
good, 27, 50, 73, 111, 114; and illness vs.
treatment removal, 97; increased risk of, 124;
inevitability of, 26–27, 30, 56, 125, 129, 142,
143, 185; and intensive care unit, 18, 49, 70;
modern definition of, 8; and natural life
span, 47–48; planning for, 180; reasoned
medical decision to allow, 96; solemn social
importance of, 29–30; states of existence
worse than, 26. *See also* dying
death panel, 30, 180
dementia, 38, 48, 82, 147, 181
diabetes, 45, 49, 152

dignity, 64, 180; and benefits vs. burdens criterion, 97; and comfort care, 18; and ethics, 68; of family, 68; of human life, 14; loss of, 111; obligation to respect, 68, 71, 72; and permanent vegetative state, 12–13
disability, 9, 19, 54, 99, 120
disease, 6, 45, 55, 110, 153–54
Do Not Attempt Resuscitation (DNAR) order, 23, 107
drug companies, 91
drugs: approval of, 182; consumer marketing of, 122; costs of, 50; diuretic, 46; erythropoietin, 152; expedited provision of, 35–36; experimental, 149; gross sales of, 152; life-ending, 135, 138; for lowering blood glucose, 152; and placebo effect, 175–76; promotion of, 46; side-effects of, 36
durable power of attorney for health care, 97, 100–101
dying: and distress from food and fluids, 132; empathy and caring, 114; and ethical intervention, 117; fear of, 129; humane and dignified, 110; prolongation of, 126, 143; special facilities for, 180. *See also* death

Elbaum, Jean, 147
Elbaum, Mr., 147
elderly people, 16, 32–33, 37, 45, 180–81; and broken hips, 57; and cost, 80, 81; death of, 34; exhaustion in care for, 54; treatment wishes of, 61. *See also* age
electronic fetal monitoring (EFM), 92
Emergency Medical Treatment and Active Labor Act (EMTALA), 165, 168, 169
empathy, 68, 70, 114
empirical evidence, 106, 139; and certainty, 105; and ethics, 158; and groups vs. individuals, 187; need for, 147–48, 153, 156; and practice guidelines, 161, 162, 166, 173–74, 179, 187–89; and predictive models, 159–60; and previous failures, 15; and public health, 154–55; research for, 141, 143; and screening, 94; and value assumptions, 174
End Stage Kidney Disease funding program, 79
Epicurus, 33–34
ethics, xi, 85, 113, 158, 176–79; and abortion, 108, 112, 176; and abuse of principles, 115; and autonomy, 81; and Baby K case, 84; and benefit, 47; and body vs. patient, 13; clarification of, 143; and comfort and dignity, 68; consultations in, 23; and encouragement to refrain from treatments, 112–14; and ends and purposes of medicine, 8; and evidence-based medicine, 154–55; and HIV infection, 108–9; and Nazi doctors, 11; and nonbeneficial treatments, 10, 51–52, 104–30; and non-citizens, 75, 76; and paternalism, 120–21, 126–27; and patient judgment, 115–19; and permanent vegetative state, 13; and permission to refrain from treatments, 111–12; and physician's judgment, 121–22; professional, 59; public education in, 142; and quality of life, 119–21, 128–29; and rationing, 82, 127–28; and religion, 122–26; and requirement to refrain from treatments, 115–18; standards for, 5, 130; and telling truth to patients, 52–53; unrealistic patient-centered, 54; and Wanglie case, 61; and withholding and withdrawing of treatment, 40
ethics committee, 145, 146
Euripedes, *Medea*, 33
euthanasia, 7, 34, 42, 133
experimental treatment, 148–50, 181–82, 188

family, 24, 25, 57–73; and adverse media attention, 35; and Alicia M., 24; approach to, 27–28; and Baby K, 41, 167; comfort of, 28, 68; communication about feelings with, 31, 32; compassion for, 13; and Cruzan, 2, 41; and decisions about care, 5; desperation of, 35; dignity of, 68; emotional support to, 20; and exhaustion of commons, 54; and fears of abandonment, 66, 70, 71, 180; feelings of, 70; loss to, 65; needs and interests of, 39; obligations of, 64–65; obligation to, 64–65; protection of, 159; refusal by, 131; and refusal to give up, 28–29; and request for treatment withdrawal, 104; rights of, 8, 131; and Wanglie, 58, 59–60, 61
family, demands of: and clear treatment standards, 165; and court cases, 41; and fear of liability, 143; increases in, 104–5; and life goals, 120; on other professions, 113, 114;

family, demands of *(cont.)*
and patient suffering, 51; reasons for, 63–65; response to, 65–68, 72–73, 100; and social values, 42; and spiritual needs, 21, 22
family planning, 54
feeding tube, 2, 3, 48; and Boxley, 52; and Mrs. Boxley, 48; and Cruzan, 3, 9; as extraordinary vs. ordinary, 97; and O'Connor, 132; and Schiavo, 41–42, 62, 63
Florida Supreme Court, 62
Food and Drug Administration, 35, 148, 149, 182
fraud, 92–93
futility, definition of, 6–14, 158, 159, 165, 169–72

Gilgunn, Catherine, 105
Grace Plaza nursing home, 147
Greeks, ancient, 6, 33, 128, 129–30, 170
guilt, 31, 64

Hafferty, Frederic, 32
Hastings Center, 40, 47, 117
Hawking, Stephen, 120
healing, 8, 10, 16, 70, 141, 143, 190
health, 10, 110, 170, 175
health care, 49; access to, 47; caps on spending in, 77; equal access to, 88; and lawyers, 91; patient-centered, 141; rationing of, 47; reform of, 45, 50, 91, 94, 128, 151, 180; rising expenditures on, 77; universal, ix
health care industry, 153, 156
health care institutions, x, 104, 176–77
health care professional, 5, 8; collaboration of, 69, 73; and commitment to patients, 141; and communication with patients, 70–71; and family demands, 63; public accountability of, 142; and standard of care, 140, 160–61; and technology, 78; values of, 11; and Wanglie case, 65. *See also* medical profession; nurse; physician
health care provider, x, 135, 159; burnout among, 53–54; communication skills and emotional sensitivity of, 68; and *ex ante* vs. *ex post* actions, 43; idealistic claims of, 147; obligation of, 13, 39, 41; psychological discomfort of, 41; standards for, 55; and Wanglie

case, 59. *See also* health care professional; nurse; physician
health care proxy, 79, 181
heart, 47, 58, 86, 158; and cardiac arrest, 17, 62, 113; disease of, 45, 49, 154. *See also* cardiopulmonary resuscitation (CPR)
heart attack, 49, 50, 79, 144, 145
Hemlock Society, 42, 116
Hennepin County Medical Center, 58, 59, 105
Hippocrates, 7, 109, 183, 190, 192
Hippocratic writings, 6, 141, 170, 173
hospice, 69, 70, 73, 180
hospital, 120; acute care, x, 18–19, 82, 106, 119, 141, 164, 175; attorneys for, 34–35, 90, 145–46; chaplain in, 124; denial of treatment by, 105; discharge from, 17, 18, 19, 50, 82, 106, 113; and Emergency Medical Treatment and Active Labor Act, 165, 168, 169; ethics committees of, 95; and fear of legal liability, 104; legal immunity of, x; and Linares, 90; and patient dumping, 165, 168, 169; and risk managers, 35; self-interest of, 146; and standard of care, xi, 16, 162, 165, 177, 185, 190–91; and technology, 4, 156; transfers from, 165. *See also* intensive care unit (ICU)
human immunodeficiency virus (HIV) infection, 55, 108–9, 177. *See also* AIDS
human life, 8, 13–14, 26, 36. *See also* person
Hume, David, 14

illness: entrapment in, 106; terminal, 82, 97, 134–35, 138, 141, 150–51, 181
informed consent, 121, 155, 156, 182, 184
insurance, 35, 47, 60, 94, 146, 154; and fraudulent treatments, 92–93; lack of, 44, 45, 116
insurance companies, 76, 154
intensive care unit (ICU), x, 4, 18, 23, 35, 117, 178, 180; and clinical predictive models, 159–60; confinement to, 19, 175; development of, 18; and extraordinary vs. ordinary treatments, 97; goal of, 49; and ineffective treatments, 52; and quality of life, 119; and Sauell case, 144, 145; time spent in, 49. *See also* hospital
Internet, 121
intubation, 52, 57. *See also* ventilator
Itami, Juzo, 30

John Paul II, 62
Jonsen, Albert R., 22
Juanita (case study), 74–76, 83, 85, 86
Judaism, 123–24, 125–26, 134. *See also* religion

Kevorkian, Jack, 34, 44, 95, 100
kidney disease, 51, 79, 97, 152

Langer, Amy, 156–57
law, x, 42–44, 102, 168, 176; and *ex ante* vs. *ex post* actions, 43; myths about, 96–101; permission vs. prohibition by, 96; and renal dialysis, 48, 49; and right-to-life activists, 206n38; and standards for legal immunity, 43; and withholding and withdrawing of treatment, 40
lawsuit, 34, 41, 57, 91–92, 95. *See also* courts
lawyer, 59, 94, 162; fear of, 91–95; representing hospital, 34–35, 90, 145–46
legal profession, 113. *See also* courts
legal surrogate, 97
legislation, 138, 164; Uniform Brain Death Act, 159; Uniform Definition of Death Act, 180; Uniform Health-Care Decisions Act, x, 164, 186
legislature, 42, 55, 62, 166, 185
liability, legal, 55, 91–92, 95, 104, 117–18, 143
life: appreciation of, 119; and awareness, emotional response, and volition, 125; and body vs. person, 9; cognitive, sapient, 97; death as accepted part of, 129; duty to preserve, 107; enhancement of remaining, 72, 73; heroic view of, 25; and human cells, 14; indefinite sustainment of, 18; intolerable state of, 25; meaning of respect for, 133–34; patient choice of qualities of, 119–20; preservation of, 14; as priceless, 50; prolongation of, 6, 7, 98, 111, 170; quality of, 9, 19, 128, 154, 158, 168; religious belief about, 124–25; right to, 13; and rudimentary state of existence, 133, 134; sanctity of, 134; sustaining of, 24; value of, 87; vitalist view of, 54, 122. *See also* biological existence; body; physiology; qualitative consideration
life support, 97, 99–100
Linares, Rudy, 89, 90–91, 147
Linares, Sammy, 89–91, 96, 99, 147

litigation: expense of, 100; fear of, 3, 91–95; and Linares, 89–91; myths about, 96–101; and Schiavo, 61–63. *See also* courts
liver disease, 49, 51
living will, 97, 99, 100–101
locked-in syndrome, 120
love, 61, 64, 65
loved one, 63, 65, 66, 100. *See also* family
Lucretius, 128–29

malpractice system, 91–92, 93
mammography, 49, 154, 156–57
media/publicity, 5, 50, 55, 84, 157, 163; and Baby K case, 84; fear of adverse, 34–35; and Linares, 90; and public judgment, 142; and Sauell case, 146
Medicaid, 60, 75, 90, 179
medical organizations, 116–17
medical paternalism, 169, 170; excessive, 52; fear of, 65, 68; potential for, 120–22; replacement of, 81; and standards of care, 126–27, 158–59
medical profession: consensus of, 180, 193; and do no harm ethic, 35, 109, 113; formulation of standards by, 121, 160–61, 165; as helping sick people, 113; moral commitments of, 110–11; and public expectations of ethical standards, 115–16; and question of money, 163; standards for, 106, 130, 139, 162; trust of, 155. *See also* health care professional; nurse; physician
medical tests, 92, 93–94
Medicare, 46, 60, 80, 180; End Stage Renal Disease Program, 48
medicine: as assisting nature, 6, 15, 141, 170; and beneficence, 11, 39; and core values, 109–11; defensive, 92, 102–3, 193; degradation of, 112; demand for, 42, 112; and discrete parts vs. whole person, 4–5; fears and inflated ideas about, 116; goals of, 138, 166, 169, 175; and healing, 16; as helping sick people, 109; hubris in, 26; integrity in, 109; junk, 92–93; and law, 91; limits of, 6, 22, 87, 117, 136, 142, 157, 172; marketing of, 71; and miracles, 29; misuse of, 47; and multiple moralities, 109; and organ systems, 9; patient-centered, 142–43; and permanent

medicine *(cont.)*
  vegetative state, 14; and prolongation of
  life, 7, 14; rational, 93; relentless faith in, 87;
  rescue, 45; as restoring health and healing
  patient, 10; source of meaning, 21; and suffering person, 14; and technology vs. patient
  care, 4; uncertainty in, 14–15, 105
metastatic cancer, 16, 107–8, 109, 113, 117, 182
Middle Ages, 6, 7, 13, 53, 170
miracle, 15, 17, 71, 95, 170, 172; and denial of
  death, 29–30; expectation of, 21–22; and
  guilt, 31; and limits of medicine, 118; and
  prayer, 118; and Tanney, 112, 113; and
  Wanglie, 58, 59
Missouri, 2–3
Missouri Supreme Court, 2
money, 44–48, 60, 77, 84, 163. *See also* cost
moral distress, 151
murder, 96–97
myth, 20, 25–26

National Alliance of Breast Cancer Organizations, 156
National Institutes of Health, 142
nature: assistance to, 6, 15, 141, 170; control
  of, 7; course of, 97; cycles of, 26; power of, 6;
  and science, 7, 170
Nazi era, 11, 127
noncitizen, 75, 76
nurse, 28; and care ethic, 68; and communication with patient, 71; and feelings, 31, 32;
  hospice, 69; intermediary role of, 122–23;
  moral distress of, 151; obligation of, 38; and
  physician, 73, 180; and religious beliefs,
  122–23; and Sauell case, 145, 151; standards
  of, 139. *See also* health care professional;
  medical profession
nursing home, 120, 180–81
Nussbaum, Martha, 25–26

Obama, Barack, ix
Obama administration, 45, 91, 151, 180
obscenity, 11
obstetricians, 92
O'Connor, Mary, 101–2, 131–35
Odysseus, 25–26, 86
Oregon, 179; Oregon Health Plan, 84

organ / organ systems, 11, 50; failure of, 50, 51,
  117, 145; transplantation of, 28–29, 77; treatment of, 145, 146; vitality of, 9

paramedics, 161
patient: abandonment of, 180; and ability to
  pay, 85; advocacy groups for, 154; and alleviation of suffering, 31; appreciation of benefit
  by, 17, 18, 19, 171; awareness of, 4–5; and
  body, 13; call to action to, 140–43; as center,
  4, 127, 136, 142–43, 146, 154, 171, 193;
  choice of, 98–99; and choice of nonbeneficial
  treatment, 118–19; and choice of qualities of
  life, 119–20; communication with, 31, 32,
  70–71, 162; and community participation,
  4–5, 19; deception of, 22, 111, 112, 178;
  dumping of, 165, 168, 169; evidence of
  wishes of, 2–3, 131–32, 134, 135; and fear
  of abandonment, 66, 67, 70, 71; feelings of,
  30, 35, 70; goals of, 169, 170; humanity of,
  66, 67; individual, 15, 75, 160, 187; information for, 22, 52, 156, 177–78; judgment of,
  121–22, 139; knowledge of, 101, 131–32,
  155–56; life goals of, 106, 175; and need for
  heroic action, 21; needs of, 11–12, 114; as
  person viewed in entirety, 70, 110, 147, 152;
  physician's relationship with, 5, 52, 66–67,
  106–7, 130, 155, 156, 177–78; psychological
  benefit to, 111; realistic expectations of,
  141–42; and relationships, 28; respect for
  choices of, 39, 41, 135–36; rights of, 8, 68,
  97, 107, 117, 182; and satisfaction from existence, 38; single vs. multiple, 85; as transfers
  from hospitals, 165; trust of, 119; understanding of, 110; as unworthy, 159; and willingness to pay, 16, 84, 128, 163; wishes of,
  58, 61, 62, 63–64, 100–102, 131–35, 140;
  worried well, 110
patient, demands of: for frivolous procedures,
  9–10; and goals, 169; increases in, 104; and
  life quality, 19; beyond limits of medicine,
  22, 42, 118; open communication about,
  100; and other professions, 113, 114; and
  right to control treatment, 53; and scarce
  resources, 82; and spiritual needs, 21
patient autonomy, 159; assistance in, 178;
  changes in, 52–53; and choice, 99; and frivo-

lous procedures, 9–10; and genuine options, 22; and goals of medicine, 19; and health care resources, 82; and medical values, 111; and nonbeneficial treatment, 188–89; and obligation of physician, 169–70; and physician authority, 39–44, 118–20; and professional standards of care, 81–83; respect for, 81; reversal of gains in, 184

Patient Self-Determination Act, 107

Patricia E. Brophy v. New England Sinai Hospital, Inc., 104

person, 147; care for, 141, 143; and medical training, 152; qualities of, 9, 12–14; relationship with, 70, 110; respect for, 87. *See also* human life

physician: abuse of power by, 121, 127, 139–40; and actions against conscience, 141; admission of failure or fault by, 31; attitudes toward telling patients truth, 52; authority of, 39–44, 118–20; and Baby K, 167, 168; and beneficence, 184; and communication with patient, 31, 32, 70–71; considered vs. negligent refusal by, 44; as counselor, 66; and courage to deny treatment, 94; and culture of silence, 92; and death of child, 32; determination of, 67–68; difficulty of refusal by, 23–26; directive to, 206n38; distraction from goals of, 114; distrust toward, 42; eighteenth-century, 110; empathy of, 68; and ethic of care, 68, 69–70, 72–73; and *ex ante* vs. *ex post* actions, 43–44; fear of lawsuits by, 34, 93, 95, 104; and fear of media attention, 34–35; flattery of, 22; as greedy, 76; and hospital attorney, 34–35; and hubris, 26; and ineffective treatments, 51–52; judgment of, 121–22; knowing use of inappropriate treatments by, 150–52; limits of, 19, 26–28, 72, 86–87; and Linares, 89–90; and malpractice system, 91–92; moral agency of, 66; moral integrity of, 112; neglect by, 159; and nurses, 73, 122–23, 180; power of, 184; and preservation of life, 107; and professional standards, 143; projection of values on patients, 155; refusal of, 24, 25, 34, 37–56, 105; and refusal to give up, 28–29; regulation of, 138, 140; relationship with patient, 5, 52, 66, 67, 70–71, 106–7, 130, 155, 156, 177–78; and resource constraints,

86; rights of, 8; and Sauell case, 145, 146; and Schiavo, 62; as self-serving, 156; social responsibilities of, 87; specialist, 145, 146–47, 153, 154; strategic concealment by, 162; trust of, 119; and Wanglie, 58, 59, 60, 61. *See also* health care professional; medical paternalism; medical profession

physician, and obligation, 19, 135; clarification of, 55; as encouraged to omit nonbeneficial therapies, 108, 109, 112–14, 177; to inform patient, 177–78; and law, 34; and miracles, 15; for nonbeneficial treatment, 41, 68, 106, 108–9, 171–72, 174; and other professions, 113–14; and patient autonomy, 188–89; and patient demands, 10, 169–70; and permanently unconscious patients, 13; as permitted to refrain from nonbeneficial treatment, 108, 109, 111–12, 176; and placebo, 118, 119, 175–76; as required to refrain from nonbeneficial treatment, 108, 109–10, 115–18, 130, 177; and suffering from nonbeneficial treatment, 51–52; to withhold treatment, 165; and younger patients, 32

physiology, 11, 14, 18; effect on, 111, 141, 143, 152; and value assumptions, 171, 186–87. *See also* biological existence; body

placebo, 118–19, 175–76

Plato, 7, 17, 18, 110, 171, 173, 175

pneumonia, 37, 38, 48, 58

poverty, 45, 116

pregnancy, 92

prenatal care, 45

President's Commission for the Study of Ethical Problems in Medicine and Biomedical and Behavioral Research, 40, 82, 113, 117

Preventive Services Task Force, 49

PRISM (Pediatric Risk of Mortality), 159

prostate cancer, 94

prostatectomy, 155–56

Protestants, 134

public: deception vs. education of, 22; demands of, 156; and demythologizing of medicine, 156; educated and active, 11; and education in ethics, 142; education of, 70; judgment of, 136–38, 140–43; knowledge of, 158

public health, 45, 154–55

Public Health Service, 142

quadriplegia, 97
qualitative consideration (quality of life), 11–12, 166; and effects on body, 164–65; and empirical knowledge, 139; parameters of, 17–20; and vegetative state, 174–75. *See also* life: quality of
quantitative consideration (likelihood of success), 11, 20, 24, 50–51, 95, 105; and empirical evidence, 163, 173–74, 188–89; and moral duty, 165; parameters of, 14–17; and placebo, 118–19; and standard of care, 166
Quinlan, Karen Ann, 95, 104, 170; and *In re Quinlan*, 95

rationing, 68, 74–88, 136, 189; appropriate invocation of, 76; and availability and cost-worthiness, 159; and costs, 77; criteria for, 85; as discriminatory, 76; and distributive justice, 75, 78, 82, 85, 116, 128; and elderly people, 81; and human limits, 86; and medical benefit, 75; necessity of, 158; and non-beneficial treatment, 80; psychological roots of, 86–88; and scarcity, 86; and self-interest, 76; and single vs. multiple patients, 85; and technology, 78; as tempered by justice, 87–88; and treatment benefit, 83–86, 127–28, 138, 157, 179, 191–92; of very-low-benefit treatments, 83
Reagan era, 54
Rehabilitation Act of 1973, 165, 168
religion, 6–7, 16, 135; and death, 25; free exercise of, 190–91; historical context of, 123, 125–26; and medicine, 21, 22; and Middle Ages, 170; and Schiavo, 62; and separation of church and state, 126; violation of beliefs in, 122–26; and Wanglie case, 58, 60; zealotry in, 3. *See also* Christianity; Judaism
renal dialysis, 48–49, 79, 97, 145, 181
resources, 77, 85, 191–92; exhaustion of, 53–54; as finite, 116; just distribution of, 179; limited, 78; squandered, 148. *See also* rationing
right-to-life activists, 99, 206n38
ritual, 21, 50, 64, 114, 172
Rome, ancient, 6, 33, 170
Rush Presbyterian St. Luke's Medical Center, 89, 90, 147

San Diego Bioethics Commission, 164
Sarah J. (case study), 28–29
Sauell, Dora (case study), 144–47, 151
Schiavo, Michael, 62, 65, 105
Schiavo, Terri, 1, 170, 206n38; and advocacy groups, 54, 99; circumstances of, 61–63; condition of, 7; divided family of, 105; feelings concerning, 64, 65; and lawsuit, 57; notoriety of, x, 41–42; and physicians, 72
Schiavo decision, 105
Schindler, Robert and Mary, 41–42, 62, 64, 105
science, 8, 78; control of nature by, 7, 170; junk, 92–93; and medicine, 68; modern, 6; objectivity in, 187; rejection of, 30; relentless faith in, 87; seventeenth-century, 13
screening, 45, 49, 94, 154, 156–57
Seattle Artificial Kidney Center, 48
Siamese twins, 50
Sibelius, Kathleen, 49
Simons, Judge, 134, 135
Sisyphus, 20–21, 86
social workers, 71
society, 138, 155; as aging, x; approval of treatment standards by, 139, 140, 160, 161, 165, 180; and beneficence, 147; consensus of, 8, 185, 193; as defining the obligations and limits of medicine, 136; education of, 166, 172; ethical role of, 106; and experimental treatments, 148, 149; formation of public judgment of, 140–43; pluralistic, 42, 190–91; and public awareness, 185; and question of money, 163; and rationing, 191; regulation by, 138, 140; as requiring nonbeneficial treatment options, 140; right to be informed, 157; values of, 8
Society of Critical Care Medicine, 40, 117, 138, 168
SOFA (Sequential Organ Failure Assessment), 159
Solomon, Mildred, 39
standard of care, xi, 8, 46, 81–82, 159; and abuse of power, 184; areas of, 140; availability of, 46, 55; and Baby K, 84, 169; and clinical practice guidelines, 153–54; debate and consensus-seeking over, 138, 166; development of, 185–86; duty to uphold, 112; establishment of, 159; formulation of, 95, 165; lack of, 55; and law, 91; and majority vs.

respectable minority standard, xi, 16, 177, 190–91; national policy for, 163; need for, 192; open discussion of, 193; public account-ability regarding, 127; publication of infor-mation about, 179, 192; public knowledge of outcomes of, 141; and scoring systems, 160, 189; social and professional approval of, 160–61; value assumptions of, 162; and Wanglie case, 59

steroids, 10–11, 16, 170

suffering/pain, 13, 38; and Alicia M., 24, 28; alleviation of, 6, 31, 38, 48, 124, 170, 180; and benefits vs. burdens criterion, 97–98; and Mrs. Boxley, 48; capacity for, 33; and CPR, 107; and expedited provision of drugs, 36; fear of, 129; freedom from, 141; hydration as adding to, 69, 98, 132; and ineffective treat-ments, 51; lessening of, 110; and medical commitment, 27; and metabolic acidosis, 69; and moral distress, 151; and nonbeneficial treatments, 94, 106, 110, 113; nutrition as adding to, 98, 132; and patient's choice of nonbeneficial treatment, 118; prevention of, 22; prolongation of, 17, 24, 28; relief of, 18, 19, 72, 114; and Tanney, 113; and trust in medicine, 155; and unrealistic legal stan-dards, 102

suicide, 7, 25, 34, 42, 96–97

Superintendent of Belcherton State School v. Saikewicz, 104

surrogate decision maker, xi, 102

Tanney, Arthur (case study), 107–9, 111, 112–13, 115

technology, 15, 17, 26, 70, 78–80; advocacy for, 156; assessment of, 154; avoidance of inva-sive, 72; and Baby K case, 84; and communi-cation about feelings, 31–32; cost of, 45, 78, 156; and defensive medicine, 103; and doc-tor-patient relationship, 87; efficacy of, 148; entrapment in, 19, 42, 67; with expanding indications, 78–79; and extraordinary vs. ordinary treatment, 97; and fear of malprac-tice suits, 93–94; and hospitals, 4; and ICU, 18; imperative of, 27; limits of, 142, 143; maintenance through, 175; marketing of, 78; misuse of, 48–52, 184–85; and need for care

standards, 169; and organ transplants, 29; and preservation of life, 13; and religion, 124; and specialists, 146–47; as symbol, 22; and termination of life support, 99; and treatment benefit, 78–79, 105–6, 140

Texas Advance Directives Act (TADA), x, 43, 186

therapy, 8, 15

tube feeding, 39–40, 79; discontinuing, x; by gastrostomy tube (case study), 38, 39; by nasogastric feeding tube (case study), 38; and other forms of treatment, 98–99; and Wanglie, 58

unconsciousness, permanent, 195n2, 196n10; and appreciation of benefits, 18; and aware-ness, 171; benefit to patient in, 175; and CPR, 161; and Cruzan, 1–3; and Linares, 89–90; and medical goals, 3; numbers of, 3; and personhood, 12; and prolongation of life, 170; and quality of life, 19, 106, 119, 141; and Schiavo, x, 1–2; and tube feeding, 79; and vitalist view, 54; and Wanglie, 57, 58, 59, 61; and Wendland, 102. *See also* brain; vegetative state, permanent

U.S. Supreme Court, 2, 39, 93, 96, 97, 99

vegetative state, permanent, 2, 7, 12, 195n2; and awareness, 171; benefit to patient in, 34, 175; and CPR, 161; and care standards, 177; defined, 195n2; and dignity and respect, 12–13; lack of experience in, 17; and moral-ity, 13; nontreatment of patients in, 117; numbers of patients in, 47; and past person, 14; and physician's ethical duty, 108; and public judgment, 141; and renal dialysis, 49, 79; and respect for life argument, 134; and Schiavo, 63; and Wanglie, 41, 57, 58. *See also* brain; unconsciousness, permanent

vegetative state, persistent, 170; and Cruzan, 3; defined, 195n2; as diagnostic entity, 3; and John Paul II, 62; and right to refuse treat-ment, 97

ventilator, 4, 50–51, 110; and Baby K, 167, 168; and criteria for death, 86; as extraordinary vs. ordinary, 97; and insurance, 35; and Linares, 89–90, 147; patient's knowledge about, 101; and quality of life, 119; and Sauell case, 144;

ventilator *(cont.)*
 and Wanglie, 57, 58, 59, 60; withholding vs.
 discontinuing, 98

Wanglie, Helga, 57–66, 72, 104–5; wishes of,
 58, 61, 105
Wanglie, Oliver, 41, 58, 59, 60, 61, 64, 65, 105

Wendland, Mrs. Robert, 102
Wendland, Robert, x, 102
withdrawal, of treatment, 40, 41, 43, 82, 98,
 100, 104
withholding, of treatment, 6, 20, 40, 82, 98,
 100, 181–82
women, 49, 69. *See also specific people*

About the Authors

Lawrence J. Schneiderman, M.D., is professor emeritus in the Department of Family and Preventive Medicine and the Department of Medicine at the University of California, San Diego, and visiting scholar in the Program in Medicine and Human Values at the California Pacific Medical Center, in San Francisco. He has been a practicing physician for more than 50 years; is founding co-chair of the University of California, San Diego, Medical Center Ethics Committee; has been an invited visiting scholar and visiting professor at institutions in the United States and abroad; and is a recipient of the Pellegrino Medal in medical ethics. Dr. Schneiderman has written more than 170 medical and scientific publications, including *The Practice of Preventive Health Care* and *Embracing Our Mortality: Hard Choices in an Age of Medical Miracles.*

Nancy S. Jecker, Ph.D., is professor in the Department of Bioethics and Humanities at the School of Medicine and adjunct professor at the School of Law and the Department of Philosophy at the University of Washington. Dr. Jecker has conducted research as a visiting scholar at the Stanford University Center for Biomedical Ethics, the Stanford University Institute for Research on Women and Gender (now the Clayman Institute for Gender Research), the Georgetown University Kennedy Institute of Ethics, and the Hastings Center. She was a visiting fellow in Princeton University's DeCamp Program in Ethics and the Life Sciences, and was twice awarded Rockefeller Resident Fellowships by the University of Texas Medical Branch Institute for Medical Humanities and the University of Maryland Center for Philosophy and Public Policy. Dr. Jecker is the editor (with Albert Jonsen and Robert Pearlman) of *Bioethics: An Introduction to the History, Methods, and Practice,* 3rd edition; and of *Aging and Ethics: Philosophical Problems in Gerontology.* Dr. Jecker has written more than 100 articles and chapters on ethics and health care.